The Silent Epidemic: Quest For A Cure

NeurAegis Drug Development For Rescuing The Brain After Concussion

Brick Tower Press
Habent Sua Fata Libelli

Brick Tower Press

bricktower@aol.com • www.BrickTowerPress.com

Library of Congress Cataloging-in-Publication Data
Baudry, Michel.
Sung, Stella M.
The Silent Epidemic: Quest For A Cure
p. cm.
1. Biography & Autobiography—Medical.
2. Medical—Neuroscience.
3. Medical—Research
Nonfiction, I. Title.
ISBN: 978-1-899694-34-1, Trade Paper

July 2025

The Silent Epidemic: Quest For A Cure

NeurAegis Drug Development For Rescuing The Brain After Concussion

Michel Baudry, Ph.D. &
Stella M. Sung, Ph.D.

AUTHORS

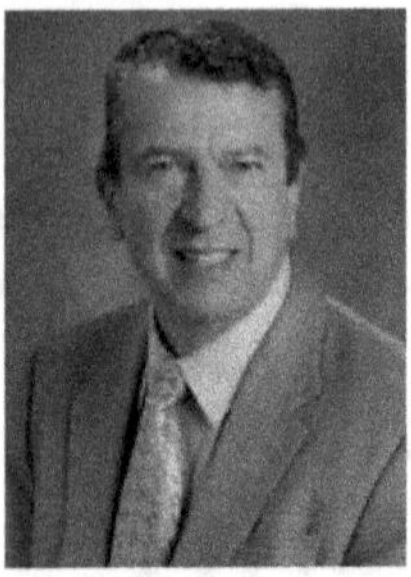

Dr. Michel Baudry

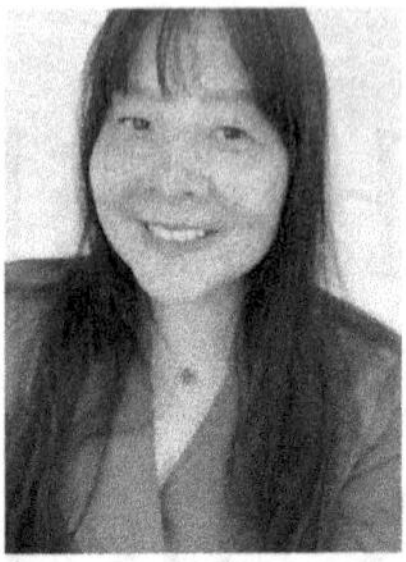

Dr. Stella Sung

"The concussion crisis has changed the face of sports as we know it and it has brought to surface the incredible importance of our brain health. The time is now for us to make our brain the number one priority so that education and awareness can take effect and begin to change the way we approach the health of our athletes from youth to professionals."

—Ben Utecht, Ambassador, The American Academy of Neurology

TABLE OF CONTENTS

OVERVIEW

Concussion is one of our most pervasive, silent epidemics. It touches many lives and often changes the course of these lives forever. Whether from sports, war, or even daily living, large swaths of our population and in the World, particularly in the elderly demographic, suffer from concussions, with an estimated >1.5 million reported concussions each year and countless more that are undiagnosed and/or unreported in the US alone. While the majority of concussions are relatively minor, many are sufficiently severe that they can result in long-term alterations in health and in some cases in death. This was exemplified in the recent movie "Concussion" starring Will Smith, which focused on the discovery and diagnosis of Chronic Traumatic Encephalopathy (CTE), particularly among football players.

Much research has been done on both the incidence and prevalence of concussion in high-impact sports such as football and hockey, even in young amateur or school age athletes. Alarmingly, it is estimated that each season an incredible 50 percent of all high school football players suffer a concussion or mild traumatic brain injury (TBI), and an estimated one-third of this group have more than one! (Source: 9 Celebrities Who Have Had Concussions | Everyday Health).

Concussions also affect those of us not engaged in high-impact sports or military combat, as we are all too often reminded by news stories of high-profile celebrities. Racing pilot Michael Schumacher suffered a terrible brain injury in a ski accident and has not been seen in public since. Derek Amato suffered a severe concussion diving in a pool and as a result became a professional piano player, although he never played piano before. Teen heartthrob Justin Bieber suffered a mild concussion during a 2012 concert in Paris, when he walked off stage, smack dab into solid glass. Bieber was "disoriented" but still managed to finish the show. However, he passed out and was unconscious for 15 seconds when he returned to his room backstage. More recently, beloved comedian and TV personality Bob Saget died suddenly at age 65 as a result of a concussion he didn't think was serious. According to his family, Saget "accidentally hit the back of his head on something, thought nothing of it and went to sleep."

These and countless other examples, including concussions that we ourselves or our friends and family may have suffered, suggest that head injuries can be significantly more serious than we think. Concussions require a more thorough understanding and new treatments that are effective and trackable.

So, what is concussion? Basically, concussion happens whenever the brain is shaken. Our brains are big gelatinous masses surrounded by three thin membrane layers, the meninges, and enclosed in our craniums. While shaking our heads in disapproval is perfectly safe, a hit on the head or an explosion nearby will produce a rapid movement of the brain that will cause it to bounce against the skull, leading to some type of damage. Generally, there are no long-term consequences, but unfortunately there are instances where this "bounce" leads to some alteration in brain structure and function. This phenomenon has been the subject of many studies and, while we have learned a lot about what happens under these conditions, we still do not have very efficient ways to protect our brains against the devastating long-term consequences of concussion.

This book will help explain what happens in the brain after concussion, but mostly this is the unfinished personal story of Dr. Baudry's dogged pursuit of finding and developing a drug capable of rescuing the brain after it suffers a concussion. The culmination of his work led to the founding of NeurAegis, Inc, a biotech company that is on path to develop new drugs that protect the brain following brain injury. NeurAegis is on the verge of initiating clinical trials for concussion with its lead drug candidate, NA-184. It is the vehicle for commercializing decades of research into treatments that have the potential to truly transform concussion care and help patients.

Research has its thrilling ups and downs, the exhilaration and despair experienced by scientists over the long periods of time required to make progress in understanding complex phenomena. The NeurAegis dream and opportunity are borne from a full five decades of research, insight and perseverance.

After earning his Ph.D. in biochemistry in the late 1970s, Dr. Baudry moved from Paris to begin research at the sunny campus of UC Irvine in Southern California. From Irvine, he went on to work for 23 years at the University of Southern California in Los Angeles. More recently, he moved to Western University of Health Sciences in Pomona, CA, where he is currently a University Professor.

Dr. Baudry's promising research has now been channeled into NeurAegis's innovative, commercially-focused vehicle. Currently, NeurAegis is achieving milestones and shaping the company's future and that of concussion patients. In the early 2020s, NeurAegis's selection of the novel molecule NA-184 to advance into the clinic was one such milestone.

The science involved is explained in a way understandable by the mainstream population and retains absolute accuracy of the facts. The science has been driving our quest since the beginning of the story; it also supports our belief that several treatments to protect the brain after concussion are on the horizon and that NeurAegis will be a key player in developing such treatments. Dr. Baudry's and ultimately NeurAegis's journey illustrates Louis Pasteur's famous assertion that "chance favors only the prepared mind", as well as Samuel Johnson's observation that "Great works are performed not by strength but by perseverance." Finding a way to treat concussions and other brain injuries is a lofty goal that is urgently needed.

Chapter 1

STARTING NEURAEGIS, INC: AN EXCITING OUTCOME OF 40 YEARS OF BASIC RESEARCH

As many a fine wine, mine and NeurAegis journey originated in France and developed and blossomed over many years. I was born and educated in France, starting from high school in Bourg-en-Bresse, a small town East of Lyon, famous for its blue-feet chicken and its cathedral. I then attended a school in Lyon that prepares students for "Les Grandes Ecoles" (a specialized university system with highly selective admission and prestigious degrees), the Lycée du Parc from 1965 to 1968. While I was there, I joined the famous "Park Glee Club", a chorus created by Professor Louis Thomas Achille and specializing in singing negro-spirituals. Our highest moment of glory took place when we were on stage when Martin Luther King visited Lyon in March 1966 and we sang with him "We shall overcome" (Fig. 1).

This was one of those moments that stay in your memory forever. Little did we know he would be assassinated 2 years later. After this school, I successfully competed to attend the Ecole Polytechnique in Paris, the French equivalent of MIT, a school established in 1794 by the

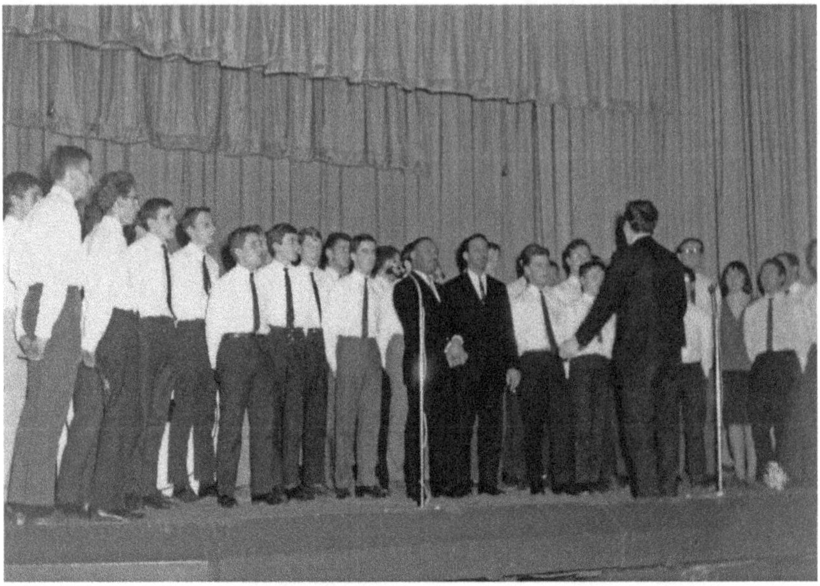

Figure 1: The Park Glee Club with Martin Luther King. Lyon, 1966.

I am the third person on the left (arrow).

mathematician Gaspard Monge[1], from 1968 to 1971. Our school motto "For Fatherland, Science and Glory", as well as the names of many famous scientists featured prominently in front of our lecture halls, served as a daily reminder of the long and famous history of the school. Throughout our three-year term, this lofty motto imprinted heavily on student minds that we were following the steps of these great scientists as well as numerous scientists and thinkers. The Ecole Polytechnique was also a great place to learn humility. After spending all my previous years at the top of each class, I was now more likely to be at the bottom of the classes, as so many of my classmates were much smarter than I was.

My almost half century career in research began in a chemistry lab at the Ecole Polytechnique. This was my introduction to the Merrifield peptide synthesis, and some 40 years later, I returned full-circle to being involved in more peptide-like synthesis[2]. The lab director, Professor Bernard Roques, encouraged his students to study biochemistry. I diligently followed Professor Roques's advice. After completing my engineering degree from the Ecole Polytechnique, I applied for a Ph.D. program in biochemistry at the University of Paris VII on the left bank of the Seine River. By then, I had already found my intellectual passion. I was committed to researching the brain and discovering the secrets of neuroscience. I was fascinated by the brain's complexity and primacy, and I was determined to use my training in chemistry and biochemistry to make significant contributions to our understanding of how this wonderfully complex mass of brain cells works.

To find a suitable laboratory and advisor for my Ph.D. studies, I visited a number of labs in France. I first spent a week in Lyon in the laboratory of Professor Michel Jouvet, famous for his work on sleep in cats. At that time, the scientists in his lab were trying to decipher the electrical patterns of brain activity responsible for the various phases of sleep, including the famous REM (rapid eye movement), which is believed to be the dream phase of sleep. I also traveled to Marseille to visit a young rising star in neurosciences, Professor Michel Lazdunski, a biochemist who has since become a world-renowned expert in ion channels. In Paris, I met with Jean-Pierre Changeux at the Pasteur Institute, a world-renowned scientist who was working on the acetylcholine receptor. One of my friends from high school and Ecole Polytechnique was already working in his lab, and as a result, Jean-Pierre did not have any openings in his lab. I also visited Professor Jacques Glowinski at the College de France, one of the founding fathers of neurobiology in France. Jacques had a large group of scientists and graduate students, and his lab was working on a group of molecules thought to be neurotransmitters/neuromodulators and called the biogenic amines, mostly dopamine, noradrenaline and serotonin. He told me that his lab was full and could not take an additional Ph.D. student, but he referred me to one of his friends, Professor Jean-Charles Schwartz, who was just starting to build a new team and was moving to a brand-new lab.

I went to talk to Jean-Charles, and he agreed to take me as a graduate student in his lab. While the new lab was being finished, I spent a few months working in Professor Schwartz's original lab in the Pharmacy of a very old hospital in Paris, the Hopital Broca, named after the famous Dr. Paul Broca. Paul Broca is best known for his work with patients with brain lesions affecting their speech, leading to the discovery of what is called the Broca area in the frontal lobe. Patients with a lesion in the

Broca area have major speech impairment. We soon moved as planned to a brand-new laboratory in a research building located next to another famous psychiatric hospital, the Hopital Ste Anne. This is where Dr. Jean Talairach developed stereotactic and functional neurosurgery, and he was still doing research on epilepsy in our building using monkeys. The animal facility in the building housed a few monkeys for his work. Once in a while, we were called to help bring monkey escapees back to their cages, which was always a frightening experience.

I spent 8 years in Jean-Charles's lab from 1971 to 1978 and my Ph.D. project was to contribute to the studies intended to demonstrate that histamine, the chemical that makes you sneeze when you have allergies, was also a neurotransmitter or a neuromodulator in the brain like the other monoamines mentioned earlier, dopamine, serotonin and noradrenaline. At the time, nobody knew what the function of histamine in the brain was, and only a handful of labs in the whole World was working on this topic. My first project was indeed very biochemistry-oriented and, together with Francois Chast, we studied the properties of an enzyme used to terminate the action of histamine, called histamine methyl-transferase. I was so happy to use all the basic biochemical analytic tools I had learned at the university to try to solve a real problem. When we were done, Francois and I wrote a manuscript, which we gave to Jean-Charles Schwartz for his approval. We were so proud of ourselves but then Jean-Charles completely rewrote the manuscript, demonstrating that writing a good manuscript requires indeed years of experience. This lesson proved to be very useful, and I have been practicing the same approach with all my trainees throughout the years. Francois Chast went on to have a brilliant career as a hospital pharmacist and has written many books, including "L'Histoire contemporaine des medicaments", and we have been friends since we first met back in 1971.

A small science society called the Histamine Club organized yearly conferences to discuss the latest findings related to the field of histamine. I met Sir James Black at one of these annual meetings. Sir Black directed a large team of scientists at Smith Kline and French (SKF), and he was awarded the Nobel Prize in Physiology and Medicine in 1988 for his contributions to rational drug design. In particular, his discovery of the H_2-histamine receptors in the stomach resulted in the development of cimetidine for the treatment of stomach ulcers. This finding led us to investigate whether these receptors were also present in the brain. Indeed, we found these receptors in the brain, and we published a manuscript reporting this discovery in the famous journal *Nature*[3]. Together with the other scientists, graduate students and technicians in the lab, we generated enough data to convince ourselves and the rest of the scientific community that histamine was indeed a neurotransmitter, as it satisfied all the criteria defining this class of signaling molecules.

Working in a lab during this period was quite different from what it is now. I remember that many people were smoking in the lab and offices, and we did not have computers and the internet. All manuscripts were first hand-written, then typed by our secretaries with typewriters; we would prepare the figures as best we could on graph paper or other support and give them to so-called graphic artists to prepare the final version we would send to the various journals we wanted to publish our papers in. There was no library in our building, and we had to request publications by sending letters to the authors of publications requesting copies or "reprints" of these articles. Alternatively, we would use Current Contents, a service database published weekly and reproducing the title pages from hundreds of journals, to find out what had been recently published.

I had minimal class requirements during the first year of graduate school and was spending most of my time in the lab running experiments. In one of the classes we had to take, and which taught me a lot, we had to read a published research article and to critically evaluate every single aspect of the manuscript. This exercise indeed demonstrated how easy it is to criticize any published work, since no manuscript is perfect. As a typical graduate student in France, I was taught that the goal of basic science is to increase our knowledge of the physical and biological world and that basic science should remain "pure" and not contaminated by its potential commercial applications. The words patent or intellectual property were not in anybody's vocabulary at the time, and it never occurred to us graduate students that there were alternatives to careers in academia or research institutes. It was made clear that the only path for our future career was to work in a university or in a research lab. I defended my thesis in 1977, and it was entitled "Histamine in the brain: Contribution to the definition of neurotransmitters." Already then, I wanted to find general principles, which would help reduce the complexity of the brain. I remained in Jean-Charles's lab for another year, until I found a lab to do a postdoctoral period. At the time, it was highly recommended for newly Ph.D. graduates to go abroad, and in particular to the United States, which was then considered to be the best place to learn the most advanced techniques, as well as to improve our speaking and writing skills in English, since English was the scientific language.

During these 8 years I learned a lot of neuroscience but also how to do research, how to ask important questions, how to design experiments and how to perform these experiments. I was lucky to be in an environment that was both friendly and intellectually stimulating. Jean-Charles had a unique style of mentoring all the lab personnel, as he was seemingly giving a lot of freedom for us to find our path, while maintaining a strict control on what we were actually doing. As mentioned above, I learned that writing a good manuscript takes a lot of practice and one needs to spend a lot of time reading the literature and writing many versions of any manuscript to make it as close to flawless as possible.

Nothing prepared me for the different paradigm and value system regarding the ultimate goals of scientific research that I encountered after moving to the US in 1978. In fact, it did not take long for me to cross the line between basic and translational science once I moved to the US.

I started my post-doctoral work in June 1978 at the University of California Irvine (UCI) in the laboratory of a young neurobiologist, Dr. Gary Lynch. At the age of 30, Gary was the second youngest full Professor in the University of California system. Gary was and still is a very unusual person, and as William Allman writes in his book "Apprentices of Wonder: Inside the Neural Network Revolution" "his intelligence and ebullient personality make him a central figure among a small group of neuroscientists who are challenging their colleagues to look beyond the strict confine of their data"[4]. He would tell all the postdocs and graduate students in the lab that he would make us "rich and famous", and that science would take care of us. Gary was working constantly, 16-18 hours a day, 7 days a week and rarely took a day off. He loved to write manuscripts in the middle of the lab while all of us were bustling about, as if he could feed on the energy to stimulate his cerebral functions. To this day, he is still working constantly and continues to make amazing contributions to neuroscience.

At UCI, I became involved in a couple of start-up companies that arose from basic research conducted in Gary's lab. In 1986, I started my science-driven entrepreneurial journey by participating in the creation of Synaptics, Inc (Synaptics). The circumstances leading to Synaptics creation reinforce the notion that life is full of surprises and that one needs to seize the opportunities that fate throws at us.

Synaptics is a company which was co-founded by Gary Lynch and Federico Faggin, the designer of the first microprocessor. The company's initial name was the Minos Corporation, from the Greek Minos, the son of Zeus and Europa, although I am not sure why Gary decided to use this name for the company. The company's ambitious initial goal was to design new computer architectures based on human brain properties. Interestingly, searching for the origin of Synaptics, Wikipedia does not list Gary Lynch (or Richard Granger or myself for that matter) as a co-founder of Synaptics[5]. Instead, it states that Synaptics was founded in 1986 by Federico Faggin and Carver Mead, who "used their research on neural networks and transistors to build pattern recognition products." In fact, it was Gary's work on neural networks that was the trigger for starting the company.

While the idea to combine knowledge on neural networks and computers was conceptually appealing, it was also too premature. At that time, computer scientists and brain scientists did not speak the same language and did not have the knowledge and the tools to merge the two fields. After one year of intense discussions between Gary and Federico and numerous trips between Irvine and San Jose, Federico renamed the company Synaptics, and he brought in Carver Mead, one of the inventors of VLSI (Very Large-Scale Integration), to develop the Human Computer Interface, starting with the famous touchpad[6]. They thanked Gary, Richard Granger and me for our contributions, but concluded that they did not need us any longer.

Several years later, the field of neurotechnologies became much more established. DARPA (the US Defense Advanced Research Projects Agency) has continued to heavily support neurotechnologies through funding. DARPA and other agencies of the Department of Defense, such as the Office of Naval Research (ONR), have been on the leading edge of developing new technologies over the last 20 years[7]. While Artificial Intelligence (AI) has been around for a long time[8], it is only recently that the field has exploded and has complemented that of neurotechnologies[9]. In addition, the Obama administration launched the Brain Initiative in 2013, a public-private initiative to develop Innovative Neurotechnologies to better understand the human brain[10]. This initiative is rapidly sprouting dozens of companies based on novel technologies. The recent advances with CHAT-GPT and the likes are another sign that the field is exploding, although the relationship of what is called Deep Learning to Human Learning is far from being obvious.

The next start-up company I was involved in, Cortex Pharmaceuticals (Cortex), was also founded in 1986 by Gary Lynch and Carol Cotman, another neuroscientist at UC Irvine. Cortex was, in part, the result of some of my experiments showing that activation of the calcium-dependent protease calpain led to neurodegeneration (more on this in later chapters). Consequently, Cortex's initial focus was the development of calpain inhibitors for the treatment of neurodegeneration. However, after several years without clear preclinical data, Cortex's strategy shifted from developing calpain inhibitors to developing different molecules that target a subtype of receptors for the neurotransmitter glutamate, which have been called ampakines[11]. Following a number of acquisitions and mergers, the ampakine program still continues under the umbrella of RespireRx Pharmaceuticals. Nevertheless, in collaboration with a chemist at Georgia Tech, Dr. Powers, Cortex generated a large number of calpain inhibitors. We took advantage of these in our search for a starting molecule for our own program at NeurAegis, Inc., some thirty years later (details in Chapter 6).

Shortly after the creation of Cortex Pharmaceuticals, I was recruited to leave UC Irvine to join a new biopharmaceutical company, Cephalon, Inc, which was co-founded in 1987 by Frank Baldino, Michael Lewis and Jim Kauer. The three founding scientists had previously worked at the giant DuPont chemical and pharmaceutical company in Philadelphia[12]. Cephalon's goal was also to develop treatments for neurodegenerative diseases. In fact, I had met Frank Baldino several times, as

Gary Lynch was a scientific advisor for DuPont and had frequent meetings with him. After a few days of soul-searching and discussions with Gary Lynch, I concluded that I was not ready to completely leave the world of academia and to move to the world of industry, especially since Cephalon was going to be located near Philadelphia. By that time, I had become a true Californian and could not see myself living on the East Coast. Interestingly, a few years later, another postdoc in Gary's lab with whom I collaborated closely, Dr. Robert Siman (aka Bob), did make the jump and went to work at Cephalon. Since he had also worked on calpains, he initiated a calpain inhibitor program at Cephalon, but this program did not lead to any drug. However, Bob ended up discovering a novel blood biomarker for TBI. This novel blood biomarker reflects the brain activation of calpain following a concussion and appears to be a good predictor for the long-term consequences of the trauma[13]. Later on, I had more interactions with Cephalon in relationship with another biotech start-up I got involved in, Eukarion, Inc., after I left UC Irvine (see Chapter 7).

I left UCI in 1989 to move to the University of Southern California (USC) in Los Angeles. A few years later in 1991, I co-founded another biotech company, Eukarion, Inc., with my very good friend, Dr. Bernard Malfroy. Bernard and I first met in Paris in 1977 when I was finishing my Ph.D. studies and he was starting his in the laboratory of Jean-Charles Schwartz. After his Ph.D., Bernard went first to do a postdoctoral period in La Jolla and then moved to Genentech in South San Francisco. Bernard and I reconnected in 1988, when I spent one year at Genentech as a visiting scientist (see Chapter 5). Bernard left Genentech in 1989 to become Director of Research in a start-up company in Boston, Alkermes[14], the same year I also left UC Irvine to take a faculty position at USC in Los Angeles. When he moved to Alkermes, Bernard and I talked about starting a calpain inhibitor program at Alkermes, but this did not materialize. After just a few years at Alkermes, Bernard decided to start his own company and he created Eukarion, Inc. Ironically, Alkermes subsequently acquired the calpain inhibitor program from Cortex Pharmaceutical but again failed to bring a calpain inhibitor to the clinic.

Eukarion's goal was to develop small molecules with enzymatic activities mimicking the enzymes superoxide dismutase and catalase, which represent the main antioxidant system in most organisms[15]. Bernard did not have a lab and asked me to be a co-founder and to use my lab at USC to launch Eukarion. The idea was exciting, and I jumped on the opportunity to start a biotech company while remaining at the university. Although we produced very compelling experimental results and published many great scientific papers, we did not succeed in raising sufficient capital to bring one of our molecules to the clinic. At some point, Cephalon offered to purchase Eukarion, but the deal did not finalize. Eukarion ended up being acquired by an Australian company in 2001, Proteome System, which never developed the Eukarion molecules, due to some strategic decisions, which took place immediately after Eukarion's acquisition. After many years of painful discussions, Bernard was able to recover the molecules from Proteome System and restarted a new company in 2008, MindSet, Rx, to continue the work with these interesting molecules. To this day, he is still working relentlessly to bring these molecules to the clinic. Interestingly, one of them (EUK-134) made it to the cosmetic industry and was initially sold by Estée Lauder. More recently, it can be found in various anti-aging products distributed by Sephora (Fig. 2).

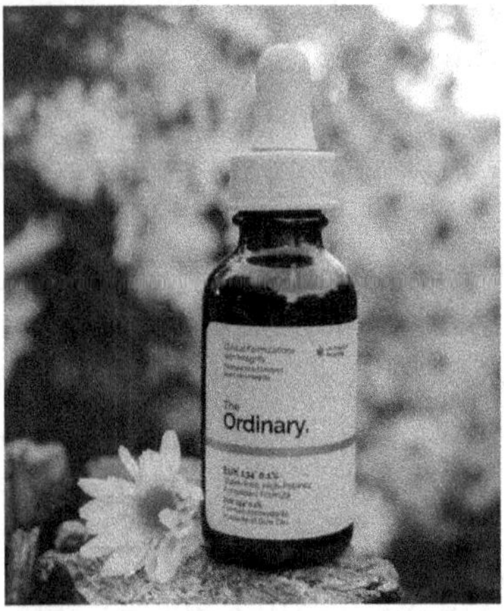

Figure 2: EUK-134 in cosmetic cream. The Ordinary EUK-134 is a serum containing the trademarked synthetic antioxidant known as Ethylbisiminomethylguaiacol manganese chloride. It mimics two enzymes naturally present in the skin, superoxide dismutase, and catalase. This means it can act as a powerful antioxidant to fights free radicals, particles that damage cells and lead to visible signs of aging, reduce redness, and protect against UV-related skin damage.

The next company I started was Rhenovia Pharma (Rhenovia), which was based in Mulhouse, France. Rhenovia's goal was to use computational neuroscience to identify new targets and new molecules to treat a variety of neurological disorders. The idea to start this company came from the work of a very talented French mathematician and medical doctor, Dr. Gilbert Chauvet, who was working with a friend and colleague at USC, Dr. Ted

Berger. The scientific community was a relatively small world at that time. I met Ted when we were both postdocs at UCI. He was working with Professor Richard Thompson, and I was working with Gary Lynch. After UCI, Ted went to work at the University of Pittsburgh. After spending several years in Pittsburg, Ted was recruited to USC by Richard Thompson. Ted's lab was just a floor above mine in the Hedco Neuroscience Building at the USC Park Campus downtown Los Angeles, next to the Coliseum. Ted and I had many discussions and ended up collaborating on several projects, as will be discussed later.

Gilbert Chauvet was a pioneer in the field of integrative biology and promoted the use of mathematics and computer science to explain complex systems, including the brain[16]. Gilbert was frequently visiting Ted at USC, and Gilbert and I had many discussions regarding his ideas to apply mathematics to understand the brain. His dream was to come up with a "simple" mathematical equation, similar to Maxwell equations, which could explain brain function. In early 2000, in collaboration with a computer scientist and entrepreneur, Dr. Yasser Al-Kazzaz, he co-founded a company called LifelikeBiomatic, Inc. LifelikeBiomatic, Inc. was focusing on using computer simulation of real neural networks to understand the effects of drugs on brain networks. Unfortunately, Gilbert died prematurely of kidney cancer, a typical example of a medical doctor misdiagnosing himself. LifelikeBiomatic did not survive without him.

In many ways, LifelikeBiomatic was the precursor of Rhenovia Pharma, which I co-founded in 2007 with another good friend of mine, Dr. Serge Bischoff. Serge was my lab coach when I started my graduate studies in the lab of Jean-Charles Schwartz in Paris in 1971. Serge taught me all the lab techniques I needed in order to work in the field of biology, since my previous lab training had been mostly in chemistry and biochemistry. We spent many hours in the lab and outside the lab when we explored a number of cheap French restaurants since we were poor graduate students. Serge left Jean-Charles' s lab in 1975 and went to work in the pharma industry, in particular at Synthelabo (which became Sanofi) in Paris and later at Ciba-Geigy, which became Novartis, in Basel, where he was project director. Serge had acquired great expertise in drug discovery and development through his industry experience. We reconnected by chance when he spent a year in La Jolla as the liaison between Novartis and the Scripps Research Institute, which was funded in part by Novartis. When Serge retired from Novartis in 2004, he settled in the South of France, near Avignon, and started a beautiful Bed and Breakfast. His Bed and Breakfast boasted a fabulous view of the Luberon, the mountain made famous by Van Gogh and other painters. When I floated the idea of starting a computational neuroscience company after Gilbert's death, Serge was enthusiastic and named our startup Rhenovia Pharma. Serge was originally from the Alsace region and had a deep knowledge of its history, closely tied with that of the Rhine River. Rhenovia was located in Mulhouse, a city on the Rhine River and in close proximity to Basel, where Ciba-Geigy's headquarters were located. Rhenovia acquired the license from USC for the use of a computer program developed in Ted Berger's laboratory. This computer program, EONS (Elementary Object of Neural System), facilitated the discovery of novel drugs or drug combinations to treat brain disorders by allowing to model the interactions of these drugs with synapses and neuronal networks. Rhenovia recruited some very talented computer scientists and a previous colleague of Serge's at Ciba-Geigy. As in my preceding startup experiences, we published many interesting papers, and we were recognized locally as an innovative company. I traveled several times a year between Los Angeles and Mulhouse, France, where we had intense working sessions with a terrific team of biologists, computer scientists and experts in drug development. We also started a US branch of Rhenovia in Boston, one of the major biotech hubs in the US, with the hope of attracting local pharma and biotech companies to our new technology. Serge even received a prestigious prize from the French Academy of Sciences[17]. While the idea was right, again the timing was not. The pharma industry was not ready for this type of approach. Rhenovia terminated its activities in 2015. Serge went back to enjoy life in the South of France, where he became and still is "a gentleman farmer." It is interesting to note that many pharma companies are now using this type of approach as well as AI technologies to facilitate drug discovery and development.

In 2012, I moved from USC to Western University of Health Sciences (WesternU), a small, private, non-profit university, located in Pomona, about 20 miles East of Los Angeles, in 2012. WesternU is about 2 miles from the famous Pomona Colleges, which include Scripps

College, Harvey Mudd College and Pitzer College. When I tell people that I work at WesternU in Pomona, most of them think that WesternU is part of the Pomona Colleges. I have to tell them that no, WesternU is not part of the Pomona Colleges, but is a small private non-profit health science university. I had been recruited as the Dean of the Graduate College of Biomedical Sciences (GCBS) and was charged to initiate a new Ph.D. program, since the GCBS only offered master programs then. I was also charged to continue my research activities as well as my company activities with Rhenovia, which I did until Rhenovia did not survive the infamous Valley of Death and terminated its operations in 2015.

One would think that after these three strikes (Synaptics, Eukarion and Rhenovia), I would have lost the desire to start yet another company. But this was not to be, and this is one of the great strengths of the American system. Failure is not a stigma but an asset and a teacher, and the ability to stand up after falling is a sign of strength and resilience, and not of weakness. I learned many lessons from these failures. In particular, that one must recognize his/her limitations, and that successful companies are built by teams of experts and not by a single individual, despite all the stories we read about Elon Musk, Bill Gates, Steve Job and the likes. Behind all of them were teams of great people who might not receive the same recognition but were essential to the success of the companies.

I also realized that I was a scientist and not a "business" person, and that I had no real interest in leading the company as its CEO. Another important lesson I learned was the necessity to be patient, as the translation from a discovery to a useful application takes a long time and is indeed like a roller coaster. One needs to have a strong stomach to survive the violent ups and downs. In other words, like basic science, translational science is not linear, and many advances are also accompanied by many setbacks. Finally, I also learned that one needs to be frugal, as money is difficult to get and whatever money is available must be used wisely.

Throughout these years and my participation in these startup companies, first in my UCI lab, then in my USC lab, and more recently in my lab at WesternU, I had continued my work to understand the roles of calpains in the brain. Importantly, almost 35 years after I started to work on calpain, I finally started to understand what these wondrous enzymes do in the brain. The critical finding was the discovery that calpain-1 and calpain-2, two calpain variants that are found in all tissues and are also called the classical calpains[18] (because they were the first members of the calpain family discovered), play opposite functions in both synaptic plasticity--the ability of synapses to modify themselves as a function of neuronal activity, and neurodegeneration--the loss of neurons following an acute insult or a slow deterioration process. Thus, calpain-1 is required for modifying synaptic function following certain types of electrical stimulation and for learning certain forms of information and is neuroprotective. In contrast, calpain-2 activation limits the extent of learning and is neurodegenerative. These findings immediately suggested to me that a selective calpain-2 inhibitor could have very broad clinical indications. Moreover, if we were right, these calpain-2 inhibitors could transform the treatment of multiple neurological disorders. To put it simply, our results predicted that a selective calpain-2 inhibitor would **facilitate learning and limit the extent of neurodegeneration** following an acute insult or trauma. Indeed, our findings in various animal tests for learning in mice and various models for acute neuronal death in mice and rats confirmed these predictions. I kept telling my students and postdocs that we had succeeded in implementing the famous pill, NZT-48, from the movie "Limitless", which in the movie expands the brain ability to learn and analyze information[19].

Although my wife and long-term collaborator, Dr. Xiaoning Bi, insisted, "You should stop wasting your time with these companies and focus on your research", I decided that I absolutely needed to start a new company to develop selective calpain-2 inhibitors as therapeutics, because universities, and especially a small university like WesternU in Pomona, do not do well these types of translational research, and are not the right place to translate a basic finding into a clinical application. Although some very large universities do have the infrastructure and the resources needed for this type of activity, WesternU was not one of these. I was undaunted by my previous entrepreneurial failures. I was convinced that our discoveries with calpain could lead to important and transformative clinical applications, and I had no choice but to start a new company. In naming the new company, I wanted to incorporate the concepts of brain and protection from damage. I thought NeuroShield could be a good name, but it had already been taken by other companies. NeuroShield is the apt product name for a brain supplement rich in antioxidants. A Canadian company was also selling a NeuroShield collar to protect athletes (mostly hockey players) from concussion—again, a well-chosen name. I then derived the name NeurAegis from the combination of Neuro and Aegis. Aegis is the Greek name for shield, as in the familiar expression "under the aegis of Zeus" from the Greek mythology. This was also a tip of my hat to Gary Lynch's Minos Corporation, as Minos was the son of Zeus.

NeurAegis, Inc. was incorporated in 2016, 30 years after starting my first company (Minos), and I was very fortunate to recruit a number of experts from my lab and my network as co-founders (Fig. 2). These experts with scientific or entrepreneurial spirit included my wife and long-term collaborator, Dr. Xiaoning Bi, another long-term collaborator from WesternU, Dr. Yubin Wang, a talented postdoc, who did most of the work on TBI and CTE, and Dr. Lina Luo, a medicinal chemist who used her skills to start working on identifying distinctive features for inhibitors of calpain-1 and calpain-2. My friends, Bernard Malfroy and an energetic entrepreneur, Greg DiRienzo, whom I had met at Western University of Health Sciences, rounded out the NeurAegis co-founder team.

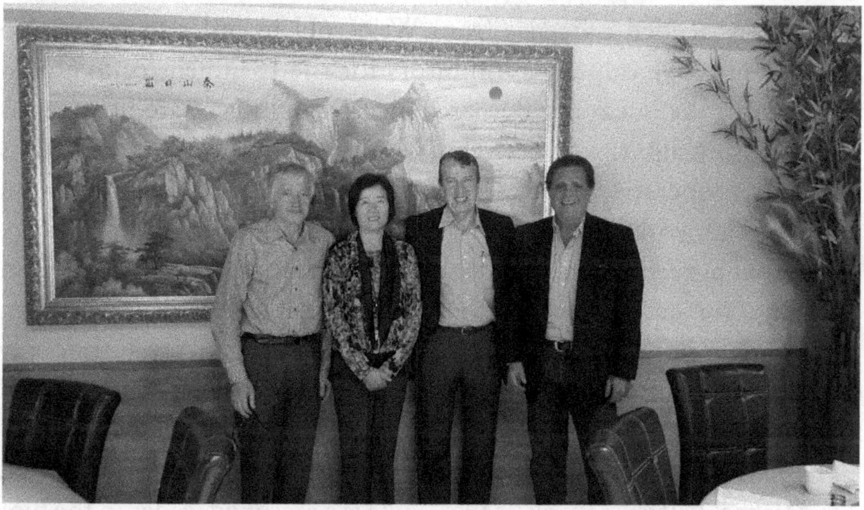

Figure 2: NeurAegis first meeting of the Board. From left to right: Bernard Malfroy, Xiaoning Bi, Michel Baudry and Greg DiRienzo.

Through Greg we worked with a talented designer who came up with the company logo, in which NeurAegis appears over what looks like a double shield (Fig. 3).

Figure 3: NeurAegis logo. NeurAegis is the fusion of Neuron and Aegis (shield), since the company is developing drugs that can protect neurons following an insult to the brain.

Starting a company is astonishingly easy, as everything can be done on-line and in a few minutes. What is hard is what follows and to put meat on the bones, and in particular to find financial support for the company activities. In my previous experiences, there was always somebody else in charge of the company who was taking care of the financial and operational nuts and bolts. This time, it was left to me and Xiaoning, and I cannot thank Xiaoning enough to put up and work with me during this early period.

Concurrently, I started filing for patents through the university tech transfer office for the discoveries and technologies my lab was producing. The university already had some experience in tech transfer as another colleague of mine had already started a company based on the intellectual property (IP) he had developed at WesternU. Next, NeurAegis needed a license from WesternU in order to be able to develop selective calpain-2 inhibitors for the treatment of neurodegeneration. We, meaning Bernard, successfully negotiated the terms of a licensing agreement between WesternU and NeurAegis. Thanks to a very cooperative VP Research, Dr. Steve Henriksen, with whom Bernard had worked when he was at the Salk Institute in San Diego, WesternU agreed to license all the IP from my lab to NeurAegis in exchange for equity in the company and future royalty payments. Upon execution of this license agreement, NeurAegis suddenly had attractive intellectual property assets as well as an experienced co-founding team.

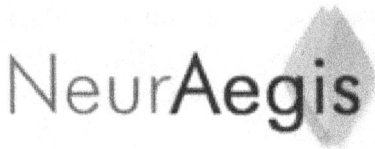

I also need to give a lot of credit to another good friend and mentor, Dr. Michael Palfreyman, aka Mike. Mike is a seasoned leader in the biotech industry, having been implicated in many small and large companies, most of them in the field of neuroscience. Our paths first crossed when he was working at Merrell Dow Laboratories and I needed some of one of the chemicals they were trying to develop, difluoromethylornithine (DFMO)[20]. He was kind enough to send me some. From then on, I always sought his advice to help with the many start-ups I was working with, and he always knew the right person to contact and talk to. When I started NeurAegis, he was an obvious choice since Merell Dow Laboratories (MDL) had a calpain inhibitor program in the 80s, out of which came a number of calpain inhibitors used in the research field even to these days. He immediately accepted to become a scientific advisor for NeurAegis and introduced me to several of his former colleagues at MDL, who had worked in the calpain inhibitor program and were delighted to become involved with NeurAegis. One of them, Dr. Philippe Bey, had a special relationship with a medicinal chemistry company in Santa Clara, Nanosyn, and after a few discussions, Nanosyn agreed to start working with us to synthesize analogs of one of the calpain-2 inhibitors we had identified from the patents published by Cortex.

The challenge then became to find funding to pay for the chemistry and for the multiple studies required by the Food and Drug Administration (FDA) before initiating clinical trials. At that time, one of the Institutes of the National Institutes of Health (NIH) had a specific program to fund the type of translational research we wanted to initiate, called the Neuroscience Blueprint Program (NBP)[21]. This program was designed to help scientists like us, who have identified a potential target for a neurological or neuropsychiatric indication and were working to discover and develop new molecules for this target. I thought that we would be ideally suited to obtain funding for this program since we already had obtained interesting preliminary data with a mouse model of traumatic brain injury (TBI).

The NIH prides itself in following a rigorous and fair evaluation process for selecting projects to fund, the so-called peer-review system. In this process, each proposal is evaluated by generally 3 reviewers who present their evaluation to a much larger panel of experts, between 20 to 30, and after 15 minutes of discussion, each member of the panel anonymously assigns a score ranging from 1 to 9. The scores are averaged, and the proposals are thus ranked from best to worst. In general, 10-12%

of the projects in a given panel end up being funded by the NIH. It is easy to see how funding is thus critically dependent on the enthusiasm, or lack thereof, for the project of 1 or 2 reviewers who have spent some time looking over the proposal. While the NIH insists on asking the reviewers not to be biased, it is also easy to see that the process is in fact extremely biased. The reviewers place a heavy weight on the names of the principal investigator (PI), the location of the PI's lab, and their potential personal connections with this PI.

To make a long story short, I submitted my project to the NBP three times and was rejected 3 times. Each time the program is reviewed, the reviewers provide the PI with a written review indicating the strengths and weaknesses of the project and justifying their scores. The main reason provided by the reviewers was that they did not believe that a selective calpain-2 inhibitor could be identified and that even if it were, it would have significant adverse effects, preventing it to ever become a pharmaceutical drug. Another reason for grant rejections was the belief by the reviewers that, since calpain had been discovered around 1960, we already knew everything there was to know about calpain. This perspective from reviewers torpedoed all my attempts for NIH funding for my calpain work, and it was difficult to counter—how do you prove what you don't know? Again, this underscores the flaws of the NIH review process. Reviews are not really based on scientific facts but on beliefs, which is quite paradoxical for scientists, and the fact is that there is very little room for real scientific innovation at the NIH. Quite interestingly, the NIH is aware of this reputational bias and is currently testing a new way of scoring proposals (https://grants.nih.gov/policy/peer/Proposed-Framework/index.htm).

Quite discouraged by these successive rejections, I turned to the Department of Defense (DoD), which had a specific call for projects for TBI. I submitted essentially the same proposal previously rejected by the NIH to the program of a branch of the DoD, the Congressionally Directed Medical Research Programs (CDMRP), which is a leader in advancing medical and scientific research by funding high impact, high risk and high gain projects that other agencies would not venture to. The proposal was well reviewed but initially not funded due to lack of funds.

However, 4 months later, I received a notification that the program was being funded because funds had become available. Funding started in July 2019, and we are now in the 4th year of the project. The goals of the project were to synthesize analogs of the selective calpain-2 inhibitor we had found in the Cortex library, to screen these molecules in in vitro and in vivo models of TBI and then select a lead clinical candidate to perform the pre-IND studies required by the FDA before being able to initiate clinical trials. We have now selected a molecule we call NA-184 and are completing the pre-IND studies and planning the Phase I clinical trial to start in 2024.

Since its creation, NeurAegis has continued to add to both the intellectual property estate and its scientific and executive team. NeurAegis has now an outstanding team of experienced drug developers, clinical and business experts who are both committed to and poised for success. More recently, Mike was also instrumental in introducing me to Dr. Stella Sung, with whom he had worked previously and whom he thought would be a great candidate for the position of CEO for NeurAegis. Stella has a prestigious background as she earned her Ph.D. in chemistry at Harvard in the lab of a Nobel Laureate. She has extensive experience as both a life science venture capitalist (VC) and an executive in various biotech companies. Mike was completely right, as Stella is now NeurAegis CEO and co-author of this book.

This book documents my long and tortuous path from being a graduate student in Paris, a post-doc at UC Irvine (who initially knew very little about neurobiology), a faculty member at three different universities, a co-founder of several biotech companies, and finally, to having the opportunity to translate all these years of research into a novel therapeutic treatment for a terrible medical condition, traumatic brain injury. The next few years will be exciting and pivotal in our goal to translate decades of research into a transformative therapeutic for the many patients who need it.

This book is also about providing information about what concussion and traumatic brain injury are and about what happens in the brain following concussion. In the process, the book will also touch upon a number of aspects of neuroscience, which were instrumental for our current understanding of the roles of calpains in the brain. This information is guiding us and other biotech companies to develop different approaches to prevent the development of brain pathologies and/or to restore normal brain function to patients suffering from concussion. And thus, a journey that began as a dream more than half a century ago in France is culminating now in the form of NeurAegis, Inc., in the fertile Southern California birthplace of many biotech startups.

Chapter 2

NEURAEGIS'S MISSION TO DEVELOP AN URGENTLY-NEEDED, FIRST-IN CLASS, TREATMENT FOR CONCUSSION & TBI PATIENTS

"Follow your heart but take your brain with you."–Alfred Adler

Concussions and traumatic brain injuries (TBIs) are both indiscriminate and commonplace. They can happen to anyone, regardless of wealth, stature, demographics, level of physical fitness or even genetics. Moreover, some concussions and TBIs have lasting and devastating consequences on health, economic, and quality of life. Some concussions and TBIs may even result in death. Perhaps the most fearsome aspect of concussions and TBIs is that they are often unpredictable, and it is not easy to determine at the time of the injury whether there will be serious outcomes. In addition to being a silent epidemic, TBI is also called the silent injury, since it often happens without the person noticing it, as discussed in a recent news story[1].

In March, 2009, famous screen and stage actress Natasha Richardson shockingly died at age 45, after hitting her head while skiing. A member of the Redgrave family and married to Oscar-winning actor Liam Neeson, Natasha Richardson was taking skiing lessons from an instructor on a beginner's trail when she fell and hit her helmetless head against the hard-packed snow at about 12:00 noon. The actress felt fine and brushed off the spill, even signing a waiver to decline medical help. A few hours later, however, Richardson had a headache and began showing signs of confusion. An ambulance took her to the local hospital and, when her situation quickly became more critical, she was transferred to a trauma center at about 6 pm that evening. Tragically, by the time Liam Neeson arrived, Natasha Richardsom was already brain-dead and on life support. Two days after the brain injury, Neeson honored their pact that if either of them were put on life support, the other would pull the plug.

In addition to Natasha Richardson, a number of high-profile celebrities and athletes have suffered concussions and brain injuries with serious consequences. Formula One legend Michael Schumacher suffered a horrific ski crash in the French Alps on December 29, 2013. He fell and hit his head on a rock, leading to a life-threatening TBI despite wearing a helmet. Schumacher was placed in a medically induced coma for 250 days. He has largely stayed at home near Lake Geneva in Switzerland and out of the public eye since being released from the hospital in 2014, and he has undergone years of further rehabilitation. The recent (2021) Netflix documentary *Schumacher* provides some family interviews and insights into both his career and his devastating brain injury.

On January 9, 2022, star of "Full House" and "Fuller House" Bob Saget died from the result of a head trauma. A statement from his family said, "The authorities have determined that Bob passed from head trauma. They have concluded that he accidentally hit the back of his head on something, thought nothing of it and went to sleep," the statement said. "No drugs or alcohol were involved."

Very recently, the NFL provided another example of the challenges facing football players when Tua Tugoveloa, the quarterback of the Florida Marlins, was carried off the field one week after receiving a concussion during the previous game. And it happened again in December, raising more questions regarding the safety of NFL players.

Concussions and traumatic brain injuries (TBI) have now been attributed to causing long-term damage and even early death in prominent athletes, as well as in many military personnel exposed to explosion and brain impact in the field. Of particular concern are injuries to the brain from repeated blows to the head or repeated blast exposure. These types of injuries can arise from tackling in football, hits and punches in boxing, or from other forceful, repeated contacts in other sports, and in professional activities. Each head injury can cause a concussion, and multiple concussions can lead to the degenerative brain condition known as Chronic Traumatic Encephalopathy (CTE), which affects many athletes.

CTE was the subject of the 2013 movie *Concussion* starring Will Smith as Dr. Bennet Omalu, the Nigerian physician who discovered CTE. The movie propelled Dr. Bennett Omalu to fame, though there have been some controversies, as reported in a recent article in the *Washington Post*[2]. In particular, Dr. Omalu's definition of CTE is now being criticized as being too broad, and his conclusion that all NFL players probably develop CTE has been refuted. It appears more likely that around 10-15% of them might develop CTE.

Examples of athletes who have suffered repeated concussions resulting in probable CTE include Kansas City Chiefs linebacker Jovan Belcher and Canadian WWE star, Chris Benoit. Both Belcher and Benoit committed murder then suicide. San Diego Chargers' hometown hero Junior Seau also committed suicide. Autopsy results showed that Seau's brain had characteristic signs of CTE. Other NFL athletes who committed suicide and were later found to have suffered from CTE include Terry Long and Dave Duerson. In fact, one could argue that there is a direct correlation between repeated concussions and depression, which in turn could lead to suicidal tendencies.

These shocking and deeply personal stories serve as everyday reminders of the very urgent medical need for an effective treatment for concussions and TBIs. TBI is the leading cause of death and disability in people age 1-44. There are about 69 million TBI cases in the World, with 2.8 million in the US and 2.5 million in Europe. Moreover, low- and middle-income countries face the highest burden with nearly three times the number of cases as high-income countries and with drastically worse neurotrauma outcomes. Of the 2.9 million people experiencing TBI each year in the USA, approximately 235,000 of them require hospitalization and 50,000 die. Those who survive often experience long-term disabilities, fatigue, depression, violence, irritability, inability to carry out day-to-day activities, and other emotional and personality changes. TBI can devastate individual lives and lives of friends and family members. Moreover, TBI imposes a heavy financial and emotional cost to our entire society.

The number of TBIs is alarmingly enormous because TBIs are caused by many factors and incidents. The most common cause of TBIs is falling with a direct hit to the head (48%). Next major causes are due to a person being struck on the head by an object or hitting the head on an object. Many athletes across different sports suffer TBIs because of this. Other TBIs result from blasts, explosions or firearms. Military personnel belong to this category because of repeated exposure to blasts and explosions. Victims of vehicle accidents often experience concussions, ranging from mild to severe. Finally, numerous concussions are due to direct personal assault. Victims of domestic violence fall into this category, although relatively few are reported. In general, concussions and TBIs are pervasive and damaging, yet significantly underdiagnosed and underreported. The urgency of addressing this "silent epidemic" is what drives NeurAegis's mission.

Currently, the diagnosis of TBI is difficult. The initial severity of the trauma is usually assessed by a series of tests evaluating certain cognitive functions, including speech, as well as the ability to control movement of eyes and limbs. These tests are part of what is called the Glasgow Coma Scale (GCS) and provide a score ranging from three to fifteen, with the lower score representing the most severe injuries. These conventional tests are arguably relatively imprecise because they rely on some qualitative evaluation and judgement. A number of companies are developing more objective tests based on biomarkers from various body fluids, including blood, saliva, urine and cerebrospinal fluid (CSF). These tests are designed to rapidly determine whether a concussion occurred and how to proceed, based on the presence and levels of specific biomarkers. The i-STAT TBI plasma test was approved by the FDA in 2018 and measures the levels of two proteins, Glial Fibrillary Acidic Protein (GFAP) and Ubiquitin carboxy-terminal Hydrolase L1 (UCH-L1)[3]. When the levels of these proteins exceed a certain value, a diagnosis of

TBI can be established. More recently, a new study provided evidence that levels of these proteins 24 h after TBI could predict the long-term outcomes from brain injury and help physicians to devise appropriate treatments for the patients[2].

Successful treatment of concussions and TBIs relies on proper diagnosis and triage. The majority of cases are mild and do not require hospitalization and do not require any treatment, beyond rest and over-the-counter pain reliever and headache medications. However, patients experiencing prolonged symptoms require some type of treatment, and the therapeutic landscape is limited. Current treatments usually target the neuropsychiatric symptoms of TBI, although new experimental treatments are directed at repairing injury, decreasing neuroinflammation, and stimulating plasticity mechanisms.

A recent Phase II clinical trial has evaluated the potential beneficial effects in TBI patients of trofinetide (NNZ-2566), a drug shown to inhibit inflammation and microglial activation in animal models of TBI[4]. However, the trial did not show a significant difference between drug and placebo in three core efficacy measures, and the development of NNZ-2566 for TBI is no longer pursued. This failure illustrates the difficulties in translating preclinical studies with good results in animal models to clinical applications in humans.

By and large, prescribed drugs today target many neurotransmitter systems, including serotonin for depression, dopamine for improved attention, acetylcholine for cognition, and glutamate for epilepsy and excitotoxicity[5]. Additional treatments target free radicals, such as N-acetylcysteine developed by Neuronasal, and nutritional supplements, although there is no clear evidence for their efficacy. Transcranial magnetic stimulation (TMS) has also been applied in TBI patients, but this technique is limited by the risk of seizures[6]. Hyperbaric oxygen treatment has also been explored with mixed results and remains controversial[7]. More recently, new approaches include Near-Infrared (NIR) therapy, stem cell therapy[8], and stimulation of neurovascular remodeling. SanBio recently completed a Phase II clinical trial in TBI patients with their proprietary stem cells, SB623 and concluded that the treatment resulted in a significant improvement of motor function[9]. In addition, new combination therapies are being tested, but these trials are not yet complete. **Currently, there are no treatments directly targeting neuronal death, a critical aspect of concussions.**

To understand the importance of neuronal death, we much understand what happens in the brain following a concussion or TBI. First, we need to define concussion. In the Oxford Language dictionary, concussion is "temporary unconsciousness caused by a blow on the head", or "a violent shock from a heavy blow." Alternatively, "concussion is a type of traumatic brain injury caused by a bump, blow, or jolt to the head or by a hit to the body that causes the head and brain to move rapidly back and forth" (CDC). It is generally accepted that there are 4 types of traumatic brain injuries: concussion, as defined above, contusion, which is a bruise on the brain tissue, penetrating brain injuries, which involve a crack of the skull and a direct hit on brain tissue, and anoxic brain injuries, when the brain does not receive enough oxygen. Another form of TBI is blast TBI, which is mostly experienced by military personnel in the field, where they are exposed to explosions that produce high energy sound waves that travel through the brain. TBI is also classified into three categories, mild TBI with either brief or no loss of consciousness, moderate TBI with a longer loss of consciousness that could last up to a few hours, and severe TBI, generally associated with crushing blows or penetration to the skull and brain and prolonged loss of consciousness.

However, this classification is not very helpful as it does not necessarily predict the long-term outcomes of the TBI. TBI includes both a very wide range of injuries and a very wide range of outcomes. This heterogeneity has been a critical challenging factor in identifying therapeutic treatments that can span the spectrum of different conditions. Experimental researchers have attempted to address the problem by developing a number of animal models for the different types of TBI, ranging from mild to severe concussion and with closed and open skull. Blast models have also been implemented in experimental animals, both in rodents as well as in non-rodents, including pigs and even monkeys. In these models, animals are exposed to blasts created in the laboratory using a variety of devices. The use of these models has produced a wealth of information and has provided the basis for starting the development of novel therapeutic approaches.

Results from experiments performed both on animal models of concussion as well as in human patients have shown that many events take place in the brain and outside of the brain and at different periods of time after the initial trauma (Fig. 1).

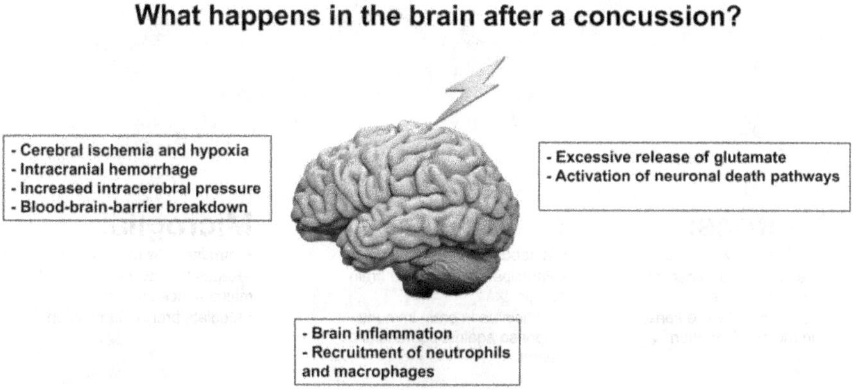

Figure 1: Schematic representation of the various events taking place in the brain following a concussion.

Before examining these post-concussion events in greater detail, we delve into the major brain cell types, which are critically involved in the pathological consequences of a concussion, i.e., neurons, astrocytes and microglia (Fig. 2).

Neurons are the basic functional units in the brain. In humans, there are approximately100 billion neurons, each of them making an average of 5-10,000 connections with other neurons. Synapses are the points of contacts between neurons. Hence, there are on the order of 1,000 trillion (10^{18}) synapses in the human brain, making it by far the most complex "object" of the universe.

While it was long considered that we were born with all the neurons we will ever possess, evidence has been accumulating over the last 20-30 years that neurogenesis, the process of generating new neurons, continues after birth and until adulthood. However, it appears that only 1,400 new neurons are generated each day and the process slows down with aging. This is indeed a very small incremental number. If this neurogenesis process would continue for about 60 years, it would only generate less than 0.03% of the total neuronal population. This also means that

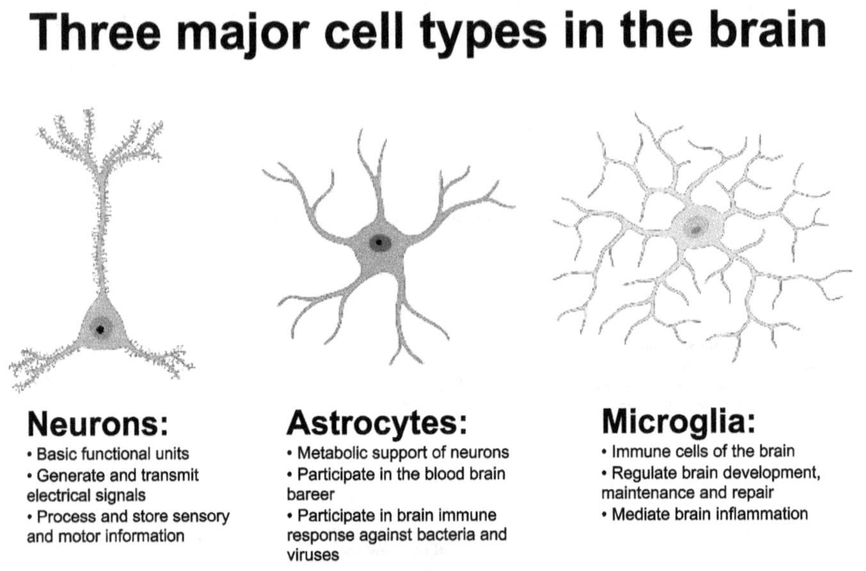
Three major cell types in the brain
Neurons:
• Basic functional units
• Generate and transmit electrical signals
• Process and store sensory and motor information
Astrocytes:
• Metabolic support of neurons
• Participate in the blood brain bareer
• Participate in brain immune response against bacteria and viruses
Microglia:
• Immune cells of the brain
• Regulate brain development, maintenance and repair
• Mediate brain inflammation

Figure 2: Three major types of cells in the brain and their functions.

Schematic representation of three types of brain cells, which play critical roles in the responses to concussions/traumas. Neurons are the cells providing for generating, propagating and transmitting information. Astrocytes are responsible for providing metabolic support but also for participating actively to immune response and maintaining the integrity of the blood-brain barrier. Microglia are the immune cells of the brain and participate in repair and inflammation.

the majority of neurons dying from insults or diseases are never going to be replaced by newly born ones.

Neurons are responsible for triggering, transporting and transmitting an electric signal, called an action potential--a brief change in the membrane potential of about 100 mV lasting 2-3 msec. It is quite remarkable that a neuron only requires 3 different proteins to produce an action potential: a sodium channel, a potassium channel, and a transporter, which exchanges sodium and potassium between the inside and the outside of the neuron.

A neuron consists of 3 cellular compartments. Like other types of cells, a neuron has a **cell body** which stores the genetic material, i,e. the DNA, and which produces most of the energy needed for function. Neurons also have **axons**, which serve as the transmitting elements--long, thin connecting structures, which originate from the cell body and end up at synaptic terminals and send electrical impulses to other neurons. The third component consist in the receiving elements of neurons, which are called postsynaptic elements and are located in **dendrites.** Dendrites also extend from the neuronal cell body, but their function is to receive, rather than transmit, messages from other neurons. Each dendrite has multiple synapses, which are contact points that connect neurons to each other (Fig. 3).

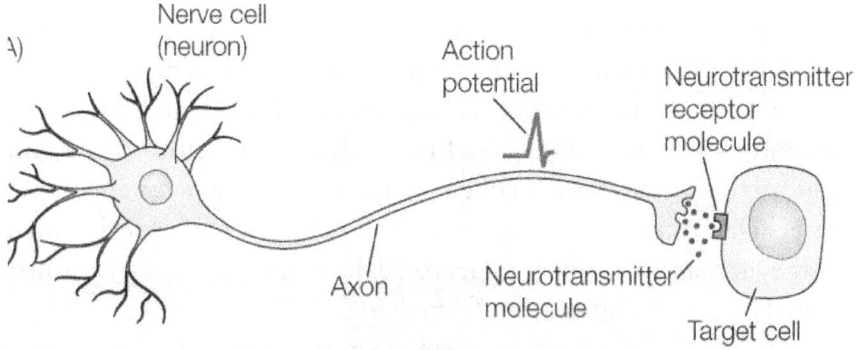

Figure 3: Basic principle of neuronal communication. An action potential is generated by the neuron, transmitted down the axon and produces the release of the neurotransmitter molecules in the synaptic terminal. The neurotransmitter diffuses across the synaptic cleft and activates receptors on the surface of the target cell. This produces either a depolarization in the case of an excitatory neurotransmitter or a hyperpolarization in the case of an inhibitory neurotransmitter. The target cell integrates all the incoming signals and either remains silent or generates an action potential that will be further transmitted.

The rate of propagation of action potentials along the axon is quite slow, ranging from less than 0.1 m/sec to 100 m/sec, and the rate of transfer of electrical signals between neurons is also very slow, between 2 and 10 msec. Clearly, these numbers pale in comparison to signal transmission in computers or cell phones, which can perform at a rate of one billionth of a second per operation. Yet, the brain still trumps the computer in solving many problems, such as identifying faces and interpreting complex images.

All sensory information is processed by specific sensors (eyes, ears, nose, tongue and skin), which transform the information (light, sound, smell, taste and pressure/temperature) into electric signals. The signals are transmitted through various networks of neurons and are integrated in sensory cortices. The content/memory of such information is stored throughout the brain. As we will discuss later, the search for the location of memories, also called engrams, dates back to Antiquity and is still a very active domain of research. In contrast, motor function is triggered by neuronal activity in the neuronal circuits that ultimately control the activities of various types of muscle types (contraction/relaxation). Thus, the loss of neurons can have multiple devastating consequences: on the receiving end of information, it can affect sensory perception (i.e., blindness or deafness), on the information processing and storing, it can result in memory loss and cognitive impairment; and on producing motor commands, it can lead to paralysis and motor impairment. Neuronal loss is the reason a concussion can have widespread and mostly irreversible functional consequences. This is why it is so critical to identify the mechanisms leading to neuronal death and to develop treatment focused on protecting neurons from dying.

For a long time, astrocytes were assumed to mainly provide metabolic support for neurons. Astrocytes are now considered to play a significantly more active role in many aspects of brain functions. They are more numerous than neurons and contribute to the regulation of synaptic transmission, water homeostasis, energy storage, and immune responses. Astrocytes are critical in establishing the blood-brain barrier, a specialized cellular complex that prevents the passage of most molecules from the blood to the brain. This barrier is essential in protecting the brain against circulating pathogens and toxins, which could cause brain infection and inflammation. The blood-brain barrier also filters the passage of selected molecules needed by the brain for normal function. While the blood-brain barrier is very beneficial, it also creates a major hurdle for delivering therapeutic drugs to the brain. Certain properties of molecules must be developed to facilitate their transport across the blood-brain barrier. As opposed to neurons, astrocytes maintain the potential to proliferate. This can also be detrimental, because uncontrolled proliferation can lead to some types of brain cancers, called glioblastoma. Most importantly, astrocytes can exist in different states. The main states are a resting state and an activated state, which is also considered to be an inflammatory state. Astrocyte activation is now related to a large number of brain disorders. In particular, astrocyte activation plays an important role following concussion.

The third type of brain cells, microglia, represent approximately 10% of the total number of brain cells and are the equivalent of circulating macrophages, cells that are responsible for the elimination of microbes and other pathogens and dead cells. In the brain, microglia are also responsible for the elimination of redundant synapses, protein aggregates and antigens that make their way across the blood-brain barrier. Microglia morphology is extremely dynamic and like the astrocytes, they exist in different states, resting and activated. They also secrete numerous pro- and anti-inflammatory molecules, called cytokines. In addition, microglia express many receptors for neurotransmitters, which indicates that they communicate with neurons, thereby regulating neuronal function. Microglia are particularly important during brain development to establish the proper organization of neuronal networks. Recent work suggests that microglia also play a critical role in brain aging. Specifically, eliminating microglia in aged mice restored cognitive functions to levels similar to those in young mice[9]. Like astrocytes, microglia are instrumental in the outcomes of many neurodegenerative diseases and following brain insults.

This background understanding of the different brain cell types provides the context for understanding the events taking place following a concussion (Fig. 1). Several events are related to changes in blood circulation in the brain. The concussion can result in the interruption of blood supply in certain parts of the brain resulting in ischemia (lack of blood supply) and hypoxia (lack of oxygen)[10]. Because both blood supply and oxygen are needed for normal cell function, lack of either one results in rapid cell damage and eventually cell death. It can also result in internal bleeding, also called intracranial hemorrhage. In turn, intracranial hemorrhage leads to increased intracerebral pressure, which activates a host of negative events, further exacerbating brain damage. Often, these events are associated with the breakdown of the blood brain barrier. Interruption of blood supply to the brain can have severe and irreversible consequences. As such, emergency personnel generally request a CT (computerized tomography) scan[11] for concussion and

TBI cases. The CT scans produce images of the brain and detect internal bleeding, blood clots, contusions and tissue swelling. These events occur early following a concussion and are generally not long-lasting if they are detected and treated rapidly. Surgery might be required to remove potential blood clots, and damaged blood vessels could be sutured to stop the internal bleeding and reduce intracranial pressure.

A concussion also triggers another series of events that is initiated by a massive release of the neurotransmitter glutamate throughout the brain. Glutamate is the major excitatory neurotransmitter in the brain. Glutamate is an amino acid that is packaged in vesicles inside neurons. These vesicles are normally released when an action potential reaches the end of the axons at the nerve endings also called synaptic terminals. When glutamate is released, it diffuses through the synaptic cleft, the small space between the synaptic terminal and the postsynaptic dendrites. Glutamate then binds to specialized receptor/channels and produces a depolarization of the postsynaptic neuron, thereby contributing to the synaptic transmission of electrical signals in the brain. Normally, glutamate is rapidly eliminated from the extracellular space by potent transport systems, which are located on glial cells and on neurons. These transport systems are specialized proteins that use energy and ion gradients to shuttle glutamate from the outside of cells to inside cells, in order to terminate synaptic transmission (Fig. 4). This is a very important step, since glutamate needs to be rapidly eliminated from the extracellular space for a new message to be transmitted from the same synapse. It is not uncommon for neurons to generate action potentials within 10 msec, which represents a firing frequency of 100 Hz, thus requiring the need for efficient transport systems. However, a concussion results in an uncontrolled and massive release of these vesicles, flooding the extracellular space with glutamate. This is often associated with the failure of the transport systems to eliminate glutamate from the extracellular space.

These events lead to the phenomenon of excitotoxicity because there is too much activation of glutamate receptors that causes uncontrolled excitation in the brain. Sometimes excitotoxicity can lead to seizure activity. In most cases, overactivation of the glutamate receptors located on the surface of neurons leads to multiple pathological events. While some of these receptors have been shown to be linked to neuroprotective

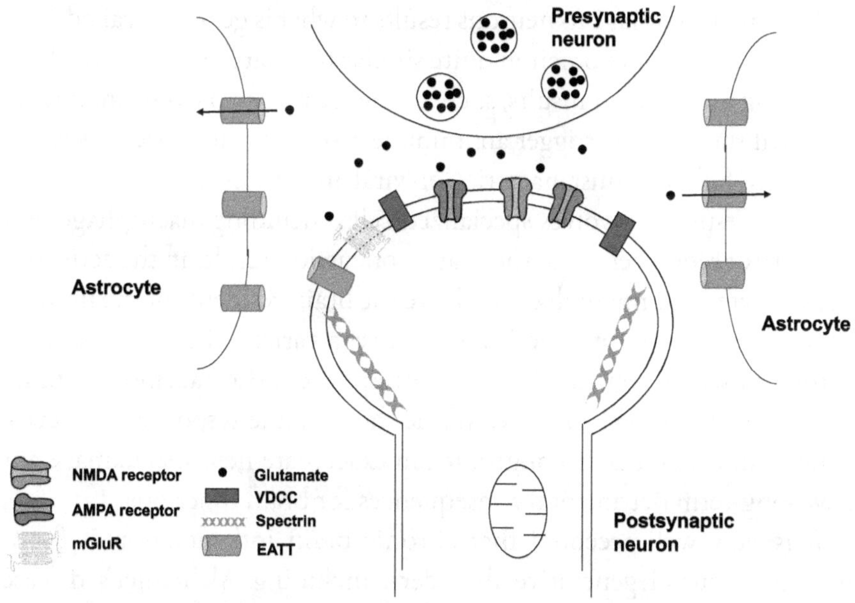

Figure 4: Schematic representation of a glutamatergic neuronal synapse, showing the release of glutamate, some of its receptors and transporters. Glutamate is stored into presynaptic vesicles and released in the synaptic cleft following an action potential in the presynaptic neuron. Synaptically-released Glu is recycled from the extracellular space by excitatory amino acid transporters (EAATs) expressed predominantly on astrocytes. Various glutamate receptors are present on postsynaptic neurons. These include both ionotropic receptors (a-amino-3-hydroxy-5-methyl-4-isoxazolepropionic acid [AMPA], N-methyl-D-aspartate [NMDA] and metabotropic receptors (mGluRs).

pathways, many are linked to neurodegenerative pathways[12]. Once the neurodegenerative pathways are activated, they can remain activated for hours, days and possibly weeks. This is one of the mechanisms that produce neuronal damage and lead to the major pathological consequences of concussion. Our work has shown that overstimulation of glutamate receptors is responsible for the activation of a calcium-dependent protease, called calpain-2, which is the major contributor to neuronal damage in the days/weeks following concussion[13]. Indeed, our studies have shown that there is a direct correlation between the activation of calpain-2 in the region surrounding the insult and the number of degenerating cells in the region[13].

In turn, the damage to neurons results in what is generally called brain inflammation, a phenomenon quite similar to what happens in the body following a number of insults, such as a bee sting or a blow to an arm or a leg[14]. All these events trigger an immune response, the process by which the body fights against bacterial or viral infections, and injuries. The immune response involves specialized cells, including macrophages and a variety of blood cells[15]. In the brain, concussion results in the activation of astrocytes and microglia, which are the brain residents of the immune system. These cells, once activated, release a variety of chemicals, called cytokines, which regulate the immune response and attract more immune cells to the site of the damage. While the immune response is generally beneficial, when it is prolonged, it can exacerbate neuronal damage and have long-term detrimental consequences for brain functions.

It is now well accepted that chronic brain inflammation is found in many neurodegenerative disorders, including Alzheimer's disease, Parkinson's disease and Amyotrophic Lateral Sclerosis (ALS, aka, Lou Gehring's disease)[16]. Several anti-inflammatory drugs, including progesterone, have been tested as potential therapeutics for TBI, but so far, none has shown clear efficacy[17]. Novel anti-inflammatory drugs are being tested both in preclinical and clinical studies.

Many potential current and future treatments for concussion are directed at interfering with neurodegenerative and inflammatory processes (Box 1).

Box 1: Drugs in the pipeline for TBI

Drug	Target	Company	Stage
PNT001	Tau antibody	Pinteon	Phase I
AST-004	Adenosine Receptor agonist	Astrocyte Pharm	Phase I
N-Acetyl-Cysteine (NAC)	Antioxidant	Neuronasal	Phase I
OXE-103	Ghrelin	Oxeia	Phase I
VAS203	Nitric oxide inhibitor	Vasopharm	Phase III
NeuroSTAT	Cyclosporin/mitochondria	Abliva	Phase II
CEVA101	Mononuclear Cells	Cellvation	Phase II
SB623	Stem cells	SanBio	Preclinical
NA-184	Calpain-2 inhibitor	NeurAegis	Preclinical

PNT001 is an antibody against the tau protein, which has been implicated in what are called tauopathies, and PNT001 been shown to have neuroprotective properties in animal models of TBI. Although the Phase I study of PNT001 was initiated in humans in 2021, the clinical trial was terminated shortly thereafter due to "administrative, non-safety related reasons." No news has surfaced since. AST-004, developed by Astrocyte Pharmaceuticals is an agonist of the adenosine receptor and has been shown to have neuroprotective properties in a rat model of TBI. N-Acetyl-cysteine (NAC) is an antioxidant and is now being developed by Neuronasal for intranasal delivery and a phase I clinical trial is being planned. Ghrelin (OXE-103, developed by Oxeia) is a gut hormone and has also been shown to facilitate recovery following TBI although its mechanism of action is not very clear. VAS203 is an inhibitor of the enzyme nitric oxide synthase, which produces nitric oxide, a modulator of blood vessel tone. It seems to have beneficial effects on several parameters measured during the Phase II and Phase III clinical trials; however, the overall functional beneficial effects do not appear to be significant[18]. NeuroStat is an analog of cyclosporin, a molecule being developed to treat mitochondrial disorders. It was developed by Abliva and reached Phase II clinical trials, but it does not look as if the company is pursuing further clinical development. CEVA101 consists of types of blood cells that have shown beneficial effects in Phase I clinical trials performed by Cellvation in 2017. However, no new results have been posted since. SB623 is comprised of another type of stem cells and is expected to undergo a Phase III clinical trial in 2024 sponsored by SanBio. It showed some beneficial effects on motor function in a Phase II clinical trial. Finally, our own NA-184 is the only drug directly targeting cell death and we are planning to initiate a Phase I clinical trial in 2024.

It would be ideal to develop a treatment that addresses all the important neurodegenerative and inflammatory processes, but this is perhaps an impossible task. The time scale of each process is different and probably varies from individual to individual. The most critical process that needs to be addressed is neuronal damage, because neuronal damage usually leads to neuronal death and permanent loss of neuronal function.

The functional consequences of such neuronal loss can vary enormously because the process could happen in many different brain regions. If neuronal damage and loss take place in the motor cortex, which is responsible for the initiation of movements, the consequences will be motor dysfunction. Neuronal damage in the sensory cortex results in sensory impairment, and language impairment is the consequence of neuronal loss in the brain regions responsible for understanding and producing language. The huge variability in functional consequences from patient to patient is indeed one of the greatest challenges in testing the effects of TBI drugs. Variability in functional consequences is also why directly targeting neuronal damage is critical. A treatment that prevents or minimizes neuronal loss will successfully treat any type of functional consequences resulting from the concussion. Moreover, preventing neuronal damage will also reduce inflammation, which arises in part from neuronal damage. NeurAegis is developing precisely this type of treatment--a drug that prevents neurons from dying after concussion. The discovery of such a drug is the product of over 40 years of cutting-edge research. It followed from Cortex Pharmaceuticals's initial goals of developing calpain inhibitors to prevent neurodegeneration. It also grew from the discovery that calpain-1 and calpain-2 play opposite functions in the brain. Finally, it has been the result of my perseverance in understanding the role of calpains in the brain and my relentless desire to translate basic findings into clinical applications.

NeurAegis's mission is to create a new class of therapeutics, selective calpain-2 inhibitors[19], which can be administered in the hours/days after injury, regardless of whether the concussion or TBI seems to be significant. Selective calpain-2 inhibitors have neuroprotective properties, as demonstrated in compelling preclinical studies done in my lab over the last 10 years. Moreover, NeurAegis's new class of therapeutics is associated with a blood biomarker that has been shown to predict the long-term outcome of TBI[20]. Practically speaking, this means that, by measuring the biomarker from a simple and painless blood test, one could immediately track and measure the effectiveness of NeurAegis's new class of therapeutics for the treatment of neurological injuries.

NeurAegis's first-in-class, trackable therapeutic could therefore transform the treatment of concussion and TBI. Decades of innovative research have created NeurAegis's opportunity to tackle an enormous unmet medical need and to make a difference in the lives of thousands and thousands of patients.

NeurAegis's and my intertwined journey spans almost a half century of relentless research. It started at UC Irvine when I was trying to understand how memories are stored in the brain. This led me to discover the roles of calpains in both learning and memory and in neurodegeneration, which subsequently resulted in the selection of a lead clinical candidate for the treatment of TBI/concussion. The quest for a cure of "the silent epidemic" spans the ups and downs of the research and discovery process and the hopes and despairs of being a neuroscientist.

Chapter 3
MY EARLY YEARS AT UC IRVINE

Like many newly minted Ph.D.s from France, I was committed to doing postdoctoral research abroad. As a graduate student in Paris, I had met a few American neuroscientists who gave me a number of suggestions and advice to identify a potential laboratory to do a postdoctoral period. It was my first exposure to the American culture and occasionally it resulted in some awkward situations. One day, an American postdoc I had met at the Ecole Normale Superieure in Paris invited me for a party at her house at 8:00pm. In Paris, this time of the day usually meant that it was an invitation for dinner. When I arrived, it was immediately very clear that this was not a dinner invitation. There were only drinks and basically no food. This was also my first-time experience at a very loud party. A lot of Americans were invited to the party, and at one point, the police showed up and asked everybody to be quiet.

Finding a lab to host me was facilitated by having already secured a position at the National Center for Scientific Research (CNRS). The CNRS is the equivalent of the National Science Foundation, while the Institut National de la Sante et de la Recherche Medicale (INSERM) is the equivalent of the NIH. A major difference between the French and the American agencies is that the French agencies do provide positions to scientists in addition to research support. I had obtained a position of Attache de Recherche, the equivalent of an Assistant Professor in an American university. This position gave me the opportunity to go abroad and still be paid by the CNRS. After being strongly advised to avoid the vast middle section of the US and jarring culture changes, I toured several labs on both the East Coast and the West Coast in September 1977. Prior to visiting labs on the two coasts of the US, I started my trip with a visit to the London lab of Sir James Black, whom I had met at the Histamine Club. At that time, he held a position at University College in London. James was very enthusiastic about me joining his lab, and I left London thinking that I had already one place to land for a postdoctoral period.

I then visited several labs on the East Coast, starting at Harvard in Cambridge. Yale and New York City were next, where I visited the labs of 2 future Nobel Laureates, Dr. Paul Greengard at Yale University and Dr. Eric Kandel at Columbia University. After a visit in Washington at a lab at St. Elizabeth Hospital, I traveled to the West Coast to labs in San Francisco, City of Hope, UC Irvine, and UC San Diego. I was extremely well received everywhere, and the lab directors, who were all very famous neuroscientists, went to great lengths to convince me to come work in their labs. My visit to UC Irvine was my first introduction to Gary Lynch and it was clearly a highlight of my trip. When I went from UC Irvine to UC San Diego, I asked some people in Gary's lab to take me to train station, as I had planned to take the train between Irvine and San Diego, as this was my usual mode of transportation in France. I was amazed to find out that most people did not know that there was a train between Irvine and San Diego, and they had no idea where the train station was. But somehow, somebody figured it out and did take me to the train station. Actually, the train ride between Irvine and San Diego is very beautiful, as the railroad follow the Pacific Coast most of the way, and I had a magnificent view of the Pacific Ocean.

I had therefore plenty of choices and needed to make a decision regarding where I was going to spend the next 2-3 years of my life. Ultimately, I was completely seduced by my visit to the laboratory of Dr. Gary Lynch at UC Irvine. I have to admit, however, that during my late September visit, I was mystified by the mass exodus occurring around

5:00pm. When I asked what was happening, people looked at me as if I was from another planet and explained that they were leaving to watch the "World Series." As a typical Frenchman, I had never heard of baseball and of the World Series—which only involves the US and Canada. I could not understand why college-educated people would sit in front of the television to watch a bunch of people chewing gum or tobacco and trying to hit a ball with a bat. Gary later spent many hours educating me on the subtleties and beauty of the sport and justifying his passion for it and for the Philadelphia Phillies, since he grew up in Delaware. Very shortly after my return to France, I told Gary that I wanted to do my postdoctoral period in his lab at UCI, thus bypassing the opportunity to do a postdoc in the lab of one of the three future Nobel Laureates I had visited (Sir Jim Black, Paul Greengard and Eric Kandel).

Looking back at my decision, there were several reasons why I chose his lab. First of all, the projects in the lab were very exciting. Gary's research was focused on trying to understand the mechanisms of learning and memory as well as those involved in brain reorganization following a lesion. Moreover, his vast cultural knowledge was amazing, and he clearly knew more about World History, literature, religion, brain evolution than anybody I had met before. Gary's attempts at speaking French with me were both pathetic and hilarious, but his energy and enthusiasm for research were contagious. The whole lab was vibrating and made me feel I would find a home there. It was also clear that Gary was interested in answering big questions regarding how the brain worked and how memories were stored and retrieved. And then, it was in Southern California, where the lifestyle was both intense, unpretentious and casual, a clear contrast with the more formal ambiance of the labs on the East Coast and even in San Francisco.

Upon learning of my carefully thought-out decision to join Gary's lab, one of my French mentors, Dr. Jean-Pierre Changeux, looked at me incredulously and said "Oh no! Gary Lynch! The hippie of neuroscience!." Indeed, Gary Lynch looked very much like Bob Dylan, and he had already acquired a reputation of being both a genius and a maverick in the field of neuroscience. When I also mentioned my decision to another American scientist working at Caltech, he told me "Don't go there, because Gary Lynch will be dead in 2-3 years, because he drinks and uses drugs!." Well, 45 years later, Gary is still around and well and working around the clock.

During the following year, when I was wrapping up my graduate work in Paris, I spent hours on the phone trying to reach Gary (the 9-hour time difference between Paris and the West Coast did not make it easy), and I was repeatedly told that he was at home writing a book. I later found out that Gary had a phobia about answering the phone and had given strict instructions to his secretary and to people in the lab, that he was not available for receiving phone calls.

Still, I arrived at UCI in June 1978, just about the time of the UCI commencement ceremony--an unfamiliar rite to a French scholar, as there is no equivalent ceremony in French universities. After participating in many graduation ceremonies in the US, I think that it is unfortunate that this tradition does not exist in France. These events do represent a very significant milestone for the students; they also strongly develop the alumni status for the graduates, which strengthens their bonds to their alma mater. These bonds have been incredibly valuable for the universities, as alumni contribute a very significant amount of the private funding for the universities.

The UC Irvine neuroscience department (actually, the department was called the department of psychobiology then) was located in Steinhaus Hall (Fig. 1) right across from the library.

It was really booming with many very talented scientists working primarily on the mechanisms of learning and memory. In particular, Professor Richard Thompson was already a leading figure in the field of neuroscience. He had just been elected a member of the National Academy of Sciences, and he led a large laboratory filled with postdocs and graduate students trying to find the famous engram, the location of a particular type of memory in the brain. As mentioned earlier, this problem dates back to Antiquity, when Greek philosophers were already intrigued by this question, which continued to keep psychologists busy throughout the 20th century.

Richard Thompson was working on a model of what is called associative learning, where rabbits are exposed to a tone and shortly after the onset of the tone, they receive an airpuff to the eye. At the beginning of the training, the rabbits close their eyes after they receive the

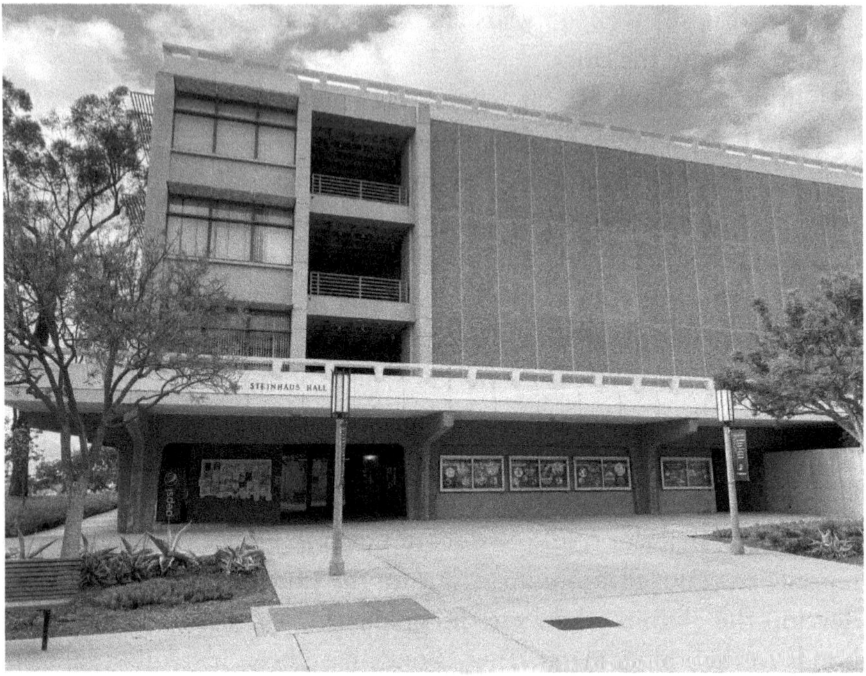

Figure 1: Steinhaus Hall on the UCI campus. Gary Lynch's lab was located right across the entry door on the first floor of the building.

airpuff. This is a reflex and the airpuff is called the conditioned stimulus (CS) giving rise to the conditioned response (CR), i.e., the closure of the eye. With training, rabbits learn to close their eyes shortly after tone onset, which is called the unconditioned stimulus (US). This associative learning model is very similar to the famous Pavlov's Dog experiments, where the dogs learned to salivate at the ring of the bell (US) because the ring had been associated with food presentation (CS). Psychologists have used and continue to use the learned US-CS associations in a large number of experiments, and US-CS association learning has been a cornerstone for the classification of various types of learning.

The first location for the engram that Richard Thompson focused on was in the hippocampus, as there was already a vast literature regarding the role of this particular brain structure in learning and memory. In particular, the notion that the hippocampus plays a critical role in human learning and memory arose from the study of a noteworthy Canadian patient, who was known for many years as H.M. (his real name was Henri Molaison), until he passed away in December 2008, and his real name was made public. H.M. was followed by two psychologists, William Scoville and Brenda Milner, who determined that H.M. amnesia was due to the ablation of the hippocampus performed by the neurosurgeon Wilder Penfield to treat his epilepsy. H.M. was quite remarkable in that he almost perfectly retained all the information he had acquired before the surgery but was unable to learn any new information of the type which is called episodic memory. Interestingly, he was still able to learn some type of information and improve in the famous cognitive test known as the Tower of Hanoi test. As a result, Scoville and Milner concluded that the hippocampus was essential to acquire new episodic information. Although initial results in the Thompson lab appeared to confirm the role of the hippocampus in learning the association between the tone and the airpuff, the experiments performed by his postdocs and graduate students after I arrived at UCI clearly indicated that the famous engram for this particular type of memory was in fact located in the cerebellum. Thus, they could make a relatively small lesion in an area of the cerebellum and completely abolish the memory trace for the US-CS association. To this day, this finding is the best example of a successful identification of a brain location for a particular memory.

While the science was exciting and stimulating, life in Irvine was a shocking contrast from life in Paris. Irvine was the home of the latest campus of the UC system, located in the heart of Orange County (OC), on land donated by the Irvine company, At the time, the campus was still surrounded by fields with happily grazing cows. Highlights of Irvine life included rodeos, drag races, and female mud wrestling, in sharp contrast to museums, classical music concerts, and theatres I was used to in Paris. People in the lab often gathered on the university baseball field on Friday afternoon, and the majority of them were pretty good baseball players. They specifically enjoyed having me on first base, as they could throw the ball as hard as they could to scare me. That's when I realized that baseball is indeed a sophisticated sport, and it is not easy to excel at it.

It took me well over 9 months to adjust to the bright, shiny newness of OC as compared to the Parisian culture I came from and to start making contributions to Dr. Lynch's research. It was also very frustrating that nobody could understand a word of what I was saying, despite my 12 years of English studies and my confidence in my English skills. It was ironic that a Polish postdoc in the lab and I had no problem understanding each other, but the native Americans standing around us could not understand anything we said. Everybody assured me that they loved my French accent, and this did not motivate me to improve my spoken English.

Culture shock was also very much evident in the lab. Shortly after I started working in the lab, I had to witness a shouting match between Gary and one of his senior postdocs. Because I was in the middle of an experiment, I could not leave the room and avoid this altercation. Coming straight from Paris, I could not believe that people in the lab could interact in such openly confrontational manner. Welcome to America! The senior postdoc later apologized for exposing me to the uncomfortable scene. He also introduced me to the hologram memory idea developed by Karl Pribram, which left a very long-lasting impression on me.

This hologram memory idea made me realized why Gary was so interested in the theta rhythm, a 5-7 Hz frequency rhythm present in the electroencephalogram (EEG), which underlies various aspects of cognitive functions and learning and memory. A hologram image is a recording of light wave interference patterns, which can be later reconstructed in 3-dimension by exposure to a coherent light wave. Thus, the hologram memory idea proposed that memories are laid down in the brain by patterns of electrical activities in various networks and retrieved when appropriate patterns of electrical activity, such as the theta rhythm, are generated in these networks.

When I joined the Lynch's lab, it was widely assumed that memories were stored in the brain by some form of activity-dependent modifications of the strength of synaptic connections between neurons. Lynch was one of the scientists who was actively studying the phenomenon of long-term potentiation (LTP), a long-lasting enhancement of synaptic efficacy elicited by brief bursts of electrical stimulation in hippocampus, a brain structure that, as mentioned above, had been implicated in learning and memory. The first manuscript reporting the existence of this phenomenon had been published in 1973 after two scientists, Tim Bliss and Terje Lomo, discovered that stimulating an input pathway with a brief burst of electrical activity in anesthetized rabbits produced a long-lasting enhancement of synaptic transmission[1]. They called this effect long-term potentiation. A great advantage of the LTP phenomenon that Gary had discovered and exploited was that it could be studied in thin slices from the rat hippocampus incubated in special dishes, where stimulating and recording electrodes could be placed at appropriate locations (Fig. 2)[2]. This made this phenomenon much more amenable to experimentation by avoiding the complexity of doing similar experiments in intact laboratory animals.

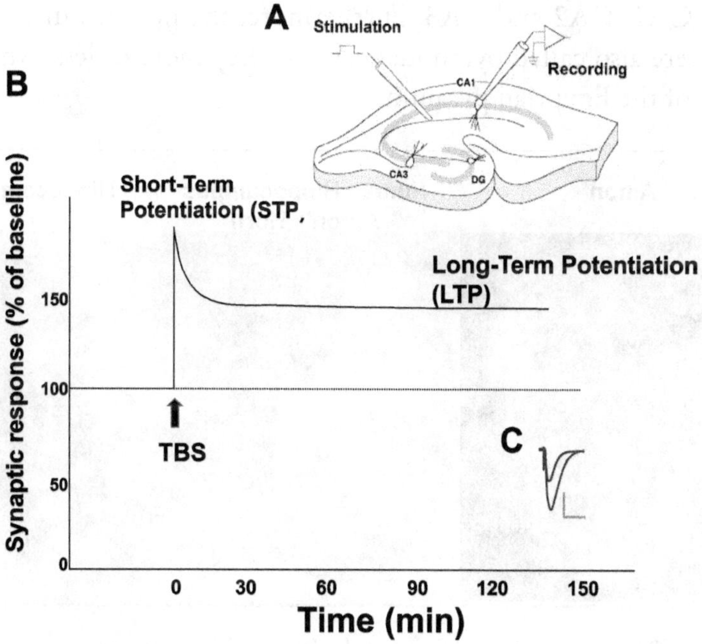

Figure 2: LTP in hippocampal slices.

A. Schematic representation of a rat hippocampal slice with recording and stimulating electrode. B. Amplitude of synaptic responses before and after delivery of theta burst stimulation (TBS). Theta burst stimulation is a pattern of brief bursts of high frequency stimulation (generally at 100 Hz) repeated at the theta frequency (5 Hz). There is an initial period of enhanced responses, which is called short-term potentiation (STP), and is followed by a stable long-term enhancement of the synaptic responses, which is called long-term potentiation (LTP). C. Examples of synaptic responses before and after TBS (Scale bars: 1 mV/5 msec).

For most people the hippocampus is a weird shape fish, which seems to stand vertically and swims by moving its tail back and forth. Why would a brain structure be called the hippocampus? As can be seen in Figure 3, the human hippocampus does look somewhat like a hippocampus. Another term for the hippocampus, which is often found in anatomy books is the Amon's horn, la Corne d'Amon (CA) in French. Again, Figure 3 explains why some anatomists in the 18th century labeled this structure the Amon' horn, as the Egyptian god Amon is often depicted with ram's horns. This analogy to the Egyptian god Amon resulted in naming various subfields of the hippocampus as fields CA1, CA2 and CA3. Furthermore, the neurons in this structure were also called pyramidal cells, as they more or less exhibit the shape of the Egyptian pyramids.

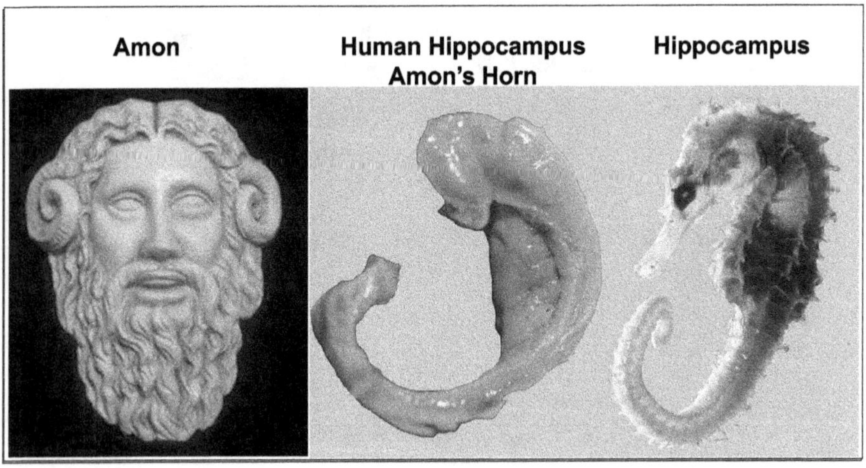

Figure 3: The origin of the name for the human hippocampus.

The human hippocampus (middle panel) received its name for its similarity to the sea creature, the hippocampus, and is also called Amon's horn for its similarity to the ram's horn, which is depicted on the head of the Egyptian God, Amon (left panel).

Because of my biochemistry background, my research focus was on finding biochemical processes that could account for the increase in synaptic transmission observed in LTP. As a graduate student I had studied a phenomenon quite similar to LTP, which we had called long-term facilitation, and this was one of the reasons I decided to do my postdoc in Gary's lab to study the mechanism of LTP. This long-term facilitation phenomenon was the result of the observation that when mice were first treated with an agonist of the receptors for the neurotransmitter dopamine, they would climb on the vertical bars of the cages they were placed in and just hang there; the length of time they were hanging was directly related to the dose of the agonist they were injected with. What we had found was that following a single injection of the agonist, a second injection resulted in a marked enhancement of the length of time the mice were hanging to the bars[3]. Hence the justification for naming this phenomenon long-term facilitation because the enhancing effects of the single injection lasted for several days. Our studies of this phenomenon pointed out to long lasting changes in the receptors for dopamine as being responsible for the enhanced responses to the second injection. In my mind, one of the most logical explanations for the enhanced synaptic transmission observed with LTP was therefore an increase in the number of the receptors for glutamate, the neurotransmitter responsible for synaptic transmission at the synapses exhibiting the LTP phenomenon. My first task was therefore to find a method to biochemically analyze glutamate receptors. In my doctoral work, I used a technique called ligand binding to study other types of receptors such as the dopamine receptors.

In this technique, one uses a radioactive molecule/ligand with a high affinity for the receptors in order to label/tag them and various methods to separate the bound from the free tag, such as filtration or centrifugation (Fig. 4).

As there were not many choices then for radioactive potential ligands to the glutamate receptors, I decided to use tritium-labeled glutamate and started to search for binding sites in synaptic membranes that could have properties of glutamate receptors.

I rapidly got the filtration technique to work and identified glutamate binding sites that had what I thought appropriate features for being potential glutamate receptors. I started publishing manuscripts reporting my findings, since publishing is the way scientists communicate their findings to the scientific community and build up their careers. At the same time, Gary's lab discovered that calcium needed to be present to

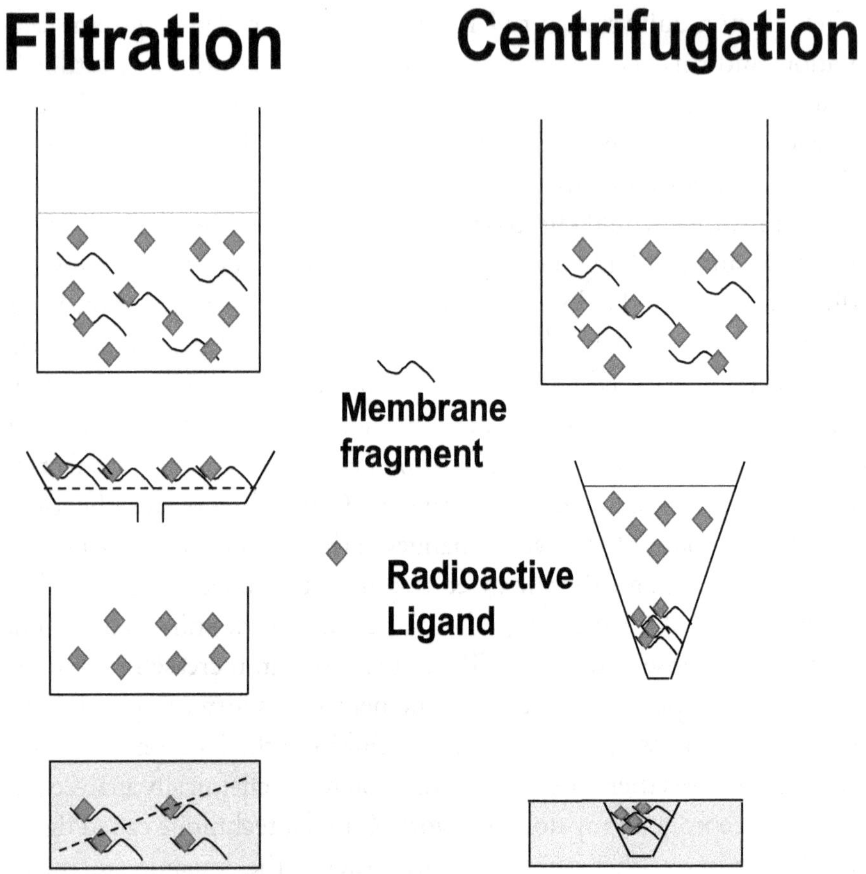

Figure 4: Two main techniques used for receptor analysis. In the filtration technique, membrane fragments are incubated with a radioactive ligand and after given time, the mixture is filtered, the filters are rapidly washed and the radioactivity retained on the filter is determined. In the centrifugation technique, membrane fragments are incubated with a radioactive ligand and the mixture is centrifuged to pellet the membrane fragments. The pellet is rapidly washed and the radioactivity remaining in the pellet is determined.

trigger the changes in synaptic strength underlying LTP[4]. I thought that it would be interesting to test whether including calcium in my binding assay could change the properties of the glutamate receptors I was measuring. Interestingly, the presence of calcium resulted in an increase in the number of receptors in the assay. Not only did calcium increase the number of receptors when present in the assay, but I could first treat the synaptic membranes with calcium and then wash out calcium and I could still measure an increase in receptor numbers[5]. This finding was quite remarkable as it indicated that calcium was acting on some elements of the membranes to produce an increase in receptors.

This served as my introduction to the world of calpain, a calcium-dependent protease, an enzyme that cleaves target proteins and modifies their functions, and which kept me busy for the next 40 + years. Calpains had been discovered in 1964, but in the 80s there were only a handful of publications reporting their properties in the brain. Most of the work had been done in Japanese labs, and notably in the lab of Dr. Murachi, which I visited a few years later. Murachi was in fact the person who changed the name of these enzymes from calcium-activated neutral proteases (CANP) to calpain, contraction of calcium and papain, a classic thiol protease (a thiol means that there is a cysteine amino acid residue participating in the active site of the protease)[6].

I was also lucky that there was another postdoc in Gary's lab who was interested in using blood platelets as a model system to investigate changes in cell structure and was working on the idea that proteases were involved in his system. He had on his shelf a number of protease inhibitors, which helped me design and run my experiments. I started to evaluate whether calpain could be responsible for the increase in glutamate receptors I found when incubating membranes with calcium. Using numerous different approaches, I did demonstrate that calpain was present in synaptic membranes[7] and, when activated, cleaved a very abundant protein in these membranes, which was called fodrin at the time[8]. Interestingly, fodrin was rapidly identified as brain spectrin, a ubiquitous cytoskeletal protein responsible for regulating cell structure by providing a mesh surrounding the cell membrane and providing both strength and plasticity to cells[9].

All of a sudden, we had discovered a mechanism that could account for many of the features we were looking at for a learning mechanism. Thus, calpain could be rapidly activated by brief periods of synaptic activity due to the resulting influx of calcium, and the resulting calpain-mediated cleavage of spectrin could lead to an increase in glutamate receptors, which would enhance synaptic strength, and also directly modify the shape of dendritic spines, the morphological substrates of synaptic communication. To further validate this idea, we showed that including a calpain inhibitor in the solution bathing the hippocampal slices blocked the induction of LTP, clearly supporting the notion that calpain activation was necessary for producing the changes in synaptic function responsible for the LTP phenomenon. This work in Gary Lynch's lab culminated with the publication in 1984 of an article in Science magazine, the top journal in the field, and to this day, this article remains a classic[10]. One of the figures from this manuscript is reproduced in Fig. 5.

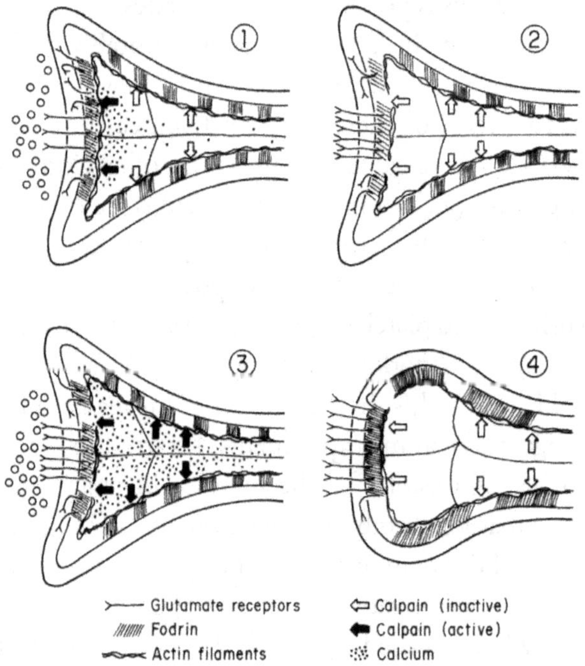

Figure 5: Schematic representation of our initial hypothesis for a learning mechanism. Activation of glutamate receptors by certain patterns of electrical activity results in an influx of calcium in the dendritic spines, which activates calpain. Calpain cleaves the cytoskeletal protein fodrin/spectrin, resulting in an increase in the number of glutamate receptors. Further activation of the process results in a modification of the structure of the dendritic spine. (Published as Figure 2 in Lynch and Baudry, Science, 224: 1057-1063, 1984. Reproduced with permission).

Gary and I were not shy, as the title of the paper was "The biochemistry of learning and memory: A new and specific hypothesis." Gary and I were ecstatic, as we really thought we had made a major breakthrough finding and provided a key piece to the puzzle of the cellular machinery underlying learning and memory. Our work caught the attention of a scientific writer for the *New York Times*, George Johnson, who came to Irvine and spent some time in Gary's lab to better understand what we were doing before writing a long article for the *New York Times*. He later further extended the story, which is reported in his book "In the palaces of memory"[11]. In this book, George explained in great detail the hypothesis Gary and I had proposed for the formation of memory, although making it clear that there were still a number of pieces of the puzzle missing. As we will see later, it took me almost 30 years to complete this puzzle.

While I was busy working in the lab, I received bad news from the CNRS. Remember that I came to the US in 1978 with my salary provided by the CNRS for 2 years. Before the end of the 2 years, I contacted the CNRS to request one more year of support since my work was going so well. Again, these communications were going through the mail since we did not have internet then. The CNRS replied that they could give me a 6-month extension. Again, at the end of the 6 months I requested another 6 months to help me finish my experiments. My request was turned down and before I could do anything I received a letter telling me that I had been fired by the CNRS. I have to say that I was somewhat shocked by this decision, which seemed so unfair considering my level of productivity during this period. Moreover, my exchange visa, which was a J-1 visa, was expiring at the end of June 1981. I had to return to Paris before this deadline in order to request a change of visa from a J-1 to an H-1 visa[12]. The UC Irvine Office of International Students was very supportive and provided the necessary documents to help me switch my visa. A critical element for the request of an H-1 visa was the approval from France of the waiver of the 2-year home requirement at the end of the period covered by a J-1 visa. I therefore went to the Ministry of Foreign Affairs to request the waiver of this requirement, since I had been fired by the CNRS. There, I was told that I should go to the CNRS in order to get this waiver. When I went to the CNRS, I was told that they did not have anything to do with me since I was no longer an employee of the CNRS. Welcome to the marvelous world of administration!

During my visit in Paris, I met several French scientists who could not believe that I had been fired by the CNRS considering all that I had accomplished in my postdoc period. They were telling me to fight back and to demand that my job was reinstated. I was caught in this strange no-man's land, since I could not, on one hand, ask for the waiver of the 2-year home requirement, and on the other hand, ask to get my job back. UC Irvine made it easier for me to resolve the problem, as I was offered a position as an Assistant Professor position in the Department of Psychobiology, although this was a non-tenure position, in the in-residence category of the UC system.

I was glad to accept this position, as it meant that I had the back-up of the UC system to resolve my visa problem. I finally got the waiver of the 2-year home requirement and was ready to switch from the J-1 to the H-1 visa. For this, I needed to go back to Paris and to have an interview at the American Embassy in Paris. Gary came along with me as he had been invited to some meetings in Europe and he walked with me to the American Embassy, although of course he could not be present during the interview. To my dismay, the Embassy employee who interviewed me rejected my application for an H-1 visa. Gary and I spent some anxious times discussing what alternatives were available for me to get the H-1 visa approved. The explanation I got for this rejection was that the interviewer was not convinced that I intended to come back to France, although the H-1 visa is used for those who intend to apply for permanent residency. I was very upset as was Gary. We called the UCI Office of International Students and explained what had happened and they indicated that they would send me additional documents to support my application. They also indicated that it would be a good idea not to return to the Paris Embassy, and that I should try to go to another location. I had an invitation to give a seminar at the Brain Research Institute in Zurich and decided to take my chance with the American consulate in Zurich. In fact, it turned out to be much easier than in Paris, as I only needed to drop all my documents on a Friday afternoon at the consulate without talking to any consulate employee. I received the famed H-1 visa in the mail on Saturday morning, which allowed me to fly back to the US on Sunday. Having resolved all these issues, I was able to continue my work at UCI. I now had my own lab adjacent to Gary's lab and I even got my own office.

After publishing our Science paper, Gary and I decided to collaborate with the lab of Richard Thompson to analyze potential changes in hippocampal glutamate receptors following learning of the US-CS association in rabbits. This was another one of these heroic experiments, which require training the rabbits for several days, and then dissecting the hippocampus out of the rabbit brain and measuring the binding of tritiated glutamate to membrane fractions prepared from the hippocampus. I had never worked with rabbits before, and it was not a small task to dissect the brain and to extract the hippocampus and prepare synaptic membranes from the large number of rabbits needed to obtain a statistically significant result. The work was mostly done by a very dedicated graduate student in the Thompson lab, who later became a Program Director at the NIH, Dr. Laura Mamounas. Along the way, like many graduate students, she did manage to make a few mistakes, which almost made me faint, such as when she miscalculated the amount of tritiated glutamate she needed to run the experiment and used almost 100 times the amount that was actually needed. But in the end, she managed to get a very interesting result indicating that indeed, binding of tritiated glutamate to rabbit hippocampal membranes was elevated following learning[13]. This was another piece of information supporting our hypothesis and showing that an increased number of glutamate receptors could be responsible for learning in other species than the rats we had been using so far.

Another significant event that took place during this period was the creation of the Center for the Neurobiology of Learning and Memory (CNLM) at UC Irvine in 1983. This Center was founded by Dr. James McGaugh, a leader in the field of learning and memory, Dr. Gary Lynch and Dr. Norman Weinberger, all World experts in this field. Richard Thompson by then had in fact moved to Stanford, which is the reason why he was not a co-founder of this Center with the other three stars of the department. It was the first research institute in the World exclusively dedicated to the study of learning and memory and I was ecstatic to rapidly become a member of the Center. Even to this day after almost 40 years, I am still and Associate Member of the CNLM. In fact, the CNLM just hosted an International Conference on Learning and Memory to celebrate its 40th birthday. The Center obtained a donation from the Bonney family, which led to the building of the Bonney Research Laboratories, and Gary and I moved our labs from the Steinhaus Hall Building in the UCI campus to this new facility in 1983 (Fig. 6). I worked there until 1989, and it was a remarkable period of intense work and great intellectual stimulation.

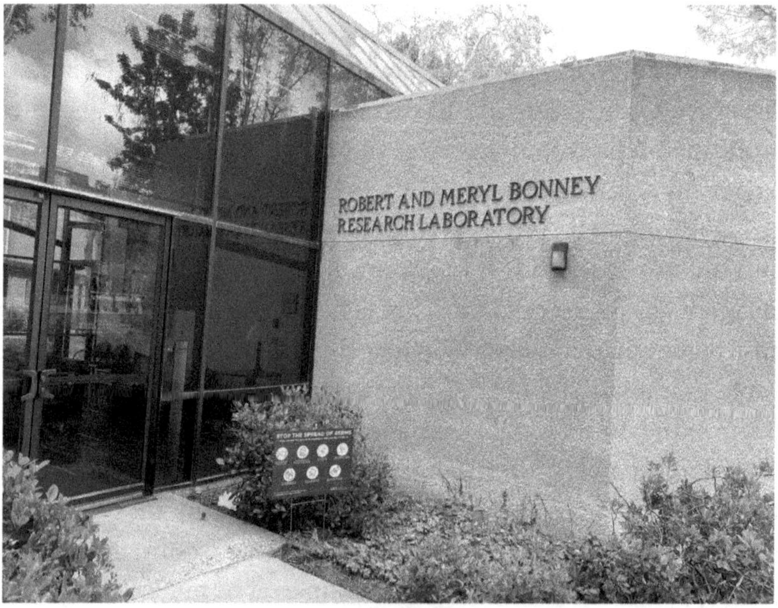

Figure 6: The Bonney Research Laboratory on the UCI Campus. It was initially called the Bonney Center for the Neurobiology of Learning and Memory when it was created in 1983 and was renamed later.

Over the years, I met many scientists who told me that the Science paper in which we proposed our hypothesis for learning and memory changed the way they understood learning and memory. Reading this paper also became a prerequisite for any student or postdoc who wanted to work in my laboratory. I also met a few scientists who thought that this publication was pure fantasy, as the experimental evidence remained relatively weak and mostly indirect. In particular, a major figure in the field recently told me "Michel, I owe you an apology. When I first read your Science paper, I thought it was pure fantasy. Now, I still think that the paper was pure fantasy, but it turned out that you were right." But it is quite typical in science that breakthrough findings are received with great skepticism and require years of additional studies before they become accepted by the majority of scientists.

Our hypothesis made the prediction that a calpain inhibitor would impair learning of certain types of information requiring the hippocampus. This was tested in two separate tasks, the so-called spatial maze (Fig. 7), in which rats have to learn which arms of the maze they have already visited to get their food reward, and an olfactory discrimination task, in which rats have to remember which odors they have been exposed to.

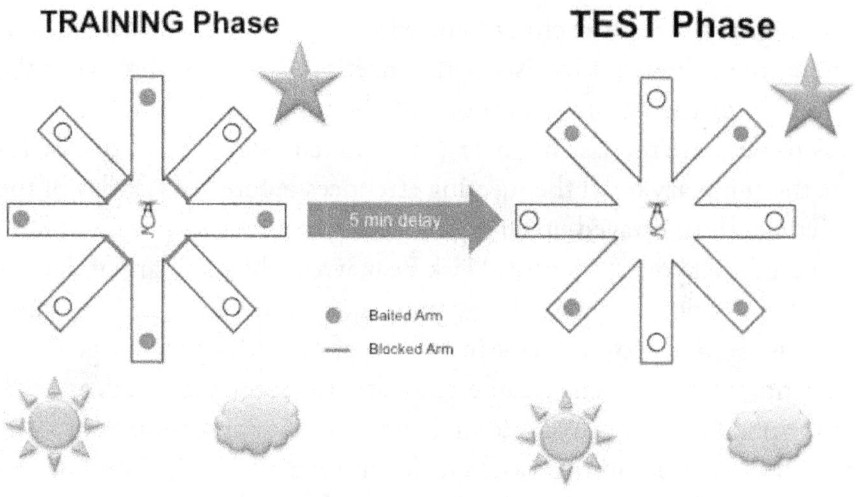

Figure 7: Schematic representation of the spatial maze.

In the training phase some of the arms of the maze are blocked and the open arms are baited with a food reward. The rats learn the location of these arms by using spatial cues in the room surrounding the maze. In the test phase, all the arms are open, and the rats have to explore those arms that were baited. Entries in the other arms are scored as errors. (from De Luca et al., 2016[14]).

In both tasks, rats treated with a relatively non-selective calpain inhibitor, leupeptin, exhibited a large impairment in learning[15,16]. On the other hand, the same inhibitor did not affect the learning of another task, avoidance learning, in which rats have to learn to avoid going to a place where they have received a foot-shock, which was known not to require the hippocampus[17]. Thus, the results of all our experiments to this point supported the hypothesis that Gary and I had proposed that calpain activation played a critical role in hippocampus-dependent learning.

These initial successes did make me relatively famous, and as a result, I was invited to a number of international conferences on the mechanisms of learning and memory where I met the leaders in the field. In particular, I was invited to a Dahlem conference in Berlin in 1985. The Dahlem conferences had been founded to stimulate multidisciplinary exchange of information on topics of international interest, and the one I had been invited to was to discuss the neural and molecular basis of learning. It was really exciting to be with the leaders of the field and, as one of the youngest scientists at the meeting, I was asked to write the summary of the discussion on one of the topics of the meeting. This was to be done the last night of the conference, as we had to distribute the summary to all the meeting attendees before the last day of the meeting. Thus, I stayed up all night writing the summary of my session while another young scientist, Mark Bear, wrote the summary of the discussion on another topic. A few years later, Mark Bear became quite famous for his discovery made in collaboration with one of his graduate students, who had been an undergraduate student in Gary's lab at UCI, of the phenomenon of long-term depression, the mirror image of long-term potentiation. In this case, a different type of electrical stimulation of inputs to the pyramidal cells of CA1 results in a long-lasting decrease in the strength of synaptic connections[18].

Chapter 4
THE HIGHER YOU CLIMB, THE HARDER YOU FALL

In the mid-80s, the scientific world started to make a dramatic turn with the advent of molecular biology and the widespread use of cloning to identify genes and novel protein families. Gene cloning is the process of identifying a particular gene by copying (cloning) it out of all the DNA extracted from certain types of cells[1]. This process allows for the sequencing, mutating and expressing the protein coded by this gene. This process was applied to identify and characterize two of the proteins our lab had been working on, the glutamate receptors and the calpains. There were already several findings indicating the existence of multiple types of glutamate receptors and of calpain variants. To identify these receptors and calpain variants, scientists used cloning, and copied the messenger RNAs present in cells into their complementary DNAs (called cDNAs) and then screening the libraries of cDNAs to find the desired proteins using what is called an expression system and an assay for the receptor or the enzyme (Fig. 1). Thus, 4 families of glutamate receptors were identified and named the AMPA, NMDA, KA and metabotropic glutamate receptors[2]. Similarly, 15 members of the calpain family (calpain-1 to calpain-15) were identified throughout the years[3], and for our work, we have focused our studies on calpain-1 and calpain-2, which are also called the classical calpains because they were the first 2 calpains identified and purified. The amino acid sequences of these 2 calpains are very similar and the major difference between these 2 isoforms[4] consists in the amount of calcium that is needed to activate them, with calpain-1 requiring very low calcium **concentration while calpain-2 requires quite high calcium concentration.**

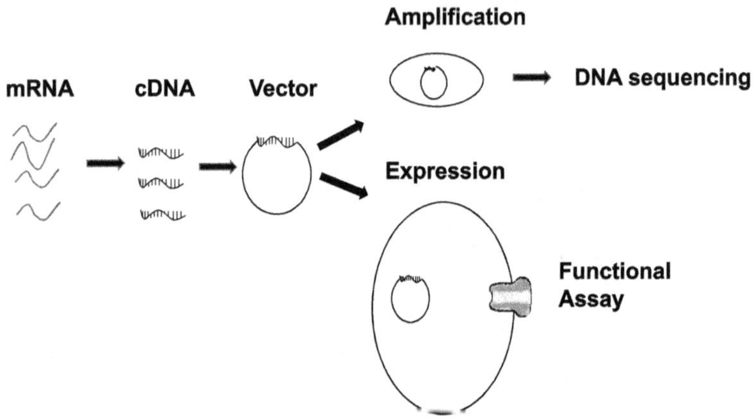

Figure 1: Cloning techniques for sequencing and functional expression.

Messenger RNAs (mRNA) from various brain regions are extracted. They are converted into complimentary DNAs (cDNA) in a test tube using various enzymes. The cDNAs are incorporated into vectors, generally small plasmids. The plasmids are amplified by incorporation in bacteria and clones containing a single type of cDNA are amplified. The DNA is then sequenced. Alternatively, the vectors are incorporated into cells, such as a frog oocyte and the protein coded by the DNA is expressed by these cells. In the case of a ionotropic neurotransmitter receptor[5], the function of this protein can be analyzed by using electrophysiology.

This later feature proved to be a serious issue, as it was not clear how this calpain variant could be activated inside normal cells, as the levels of calcium could never reach such high values. Consequently, most researchers in the field have assumed that calpain-1 was the isoform responsible for carrying out most calpain functions in the brain. It is important to stress that while molecular biology has allowed the cloning and characterization of 15 different genes and therefore 15 different types of calpains, we still know very little about each of these 15 different calpains.

Some of them are ubiquitous, meaning that they are found in most cells and tissues (this is the case for calpain-1 and calpain-2), others have a very selective distribution in certain cell types and organs. We also know now that mutations in some of the genes coding for certain types of calpains are involved in certain diseases. This is particularly the case for calpain-3, which is found predominantly in muscles and when mutated produces a form of muscular dystrophy called limb girdle muscular dystrophy (LGMD)[6]. But for the majority of the calpain variants, we still know very little about their functions, their protein targets, and their regulation. We recently reviewed the state of our knowledge on calpains, which illustrate both the progress made since the initial discovery but also all the gaps in our knowledge of this clearly very important class of enzymes[3]. To this day, I am still dumbfounded that not much effort is being devoted to fill these gaps. Every time I have submitted a grant application to the NIH to answer critical questions related to calpain, the reviewers turned them down by saying that everything was known on calpain...

The atmosphere at UCI in the early 80s was intensely competitive, as the department of psychobiology where Gary was a faculty had been built by a few senior scientists and several junior scientists, who already were or rapidly were becoming leaders in the field of neuroscience. In particular, there was some overlap in the work on glutamate receptors between the laboratories of Gary Lynch and Carl Cotman, two of the bright young stars of the department, which made life more complicated for the postdocs working in their labs, as there was an implicit rule to minimize scientific communication between the two laboratories. I remember running into a postdoc from the Cotman lab in the copy room, and it was quite odd, as we were both hiding whatever we were making copies of.

This became especially important after the discovery and characterization of one subtype of glutamate receptors, the so-called NMDA receptor. This receptor has the remarkable property of being responsive to the neurotransmitter glutamate only when the membrane is depolarized, making it an ideal candidate for participating in learning and memory, since it exhibits a clear associative property, meaning that two items are linked together, which scientists believed to be an essential property of learning, as discussed above in the rabbit experiments. In other words, the NMDA receptor is only activated when two events are taking place, a release of glutamate from the presynaptic terminal, and the postsynaptic membrane is depolarized. The reason for this was also explained when it was found out that under basal conditions, i.e., when the membrane was at the resting negative potential, magnesium was blocking the ion channel formed by the subunits of the NMDA receptor[7] (Fig. 2). For computer scientists, this receptor therefore functions as an AND gate. Of course, the idea that NMDA receptors were critical for learning needed to be verified experimentally.

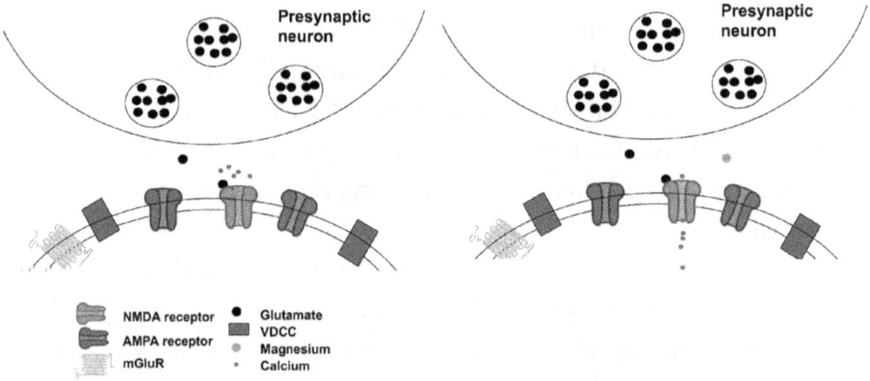

Figure 2. Schematic representation of the function of the NMDA receptor.

Left: under basal conditions, magnesium ions block the NMDA receptor/channel. Even if glutamate is released from the presynaptic terminal and binds to the receptor, no current is generated by the receptor. Right: if the postsynaptic membrane is depolarized, magnesium ions are ejected from the NMDA receptor/channel and the release of glutamate from the presynaptic terminal results in the activation of the NMDA receptors and the generation of a postsynaptic response and an influx of calcium in the postsynaptic terminal.

The Lynch lab effectively won the competition when Richard Morris visited UC Irvine for one of the International Conference on Learning and Memory that the CNLM regularly organized (Fig. 3). These conferences were the opportunity for scientists from all over the World to gather and discuss the latest findings in their field. They were also providing them the opportunity to initiate collaborative projects to test specific hypothesis.

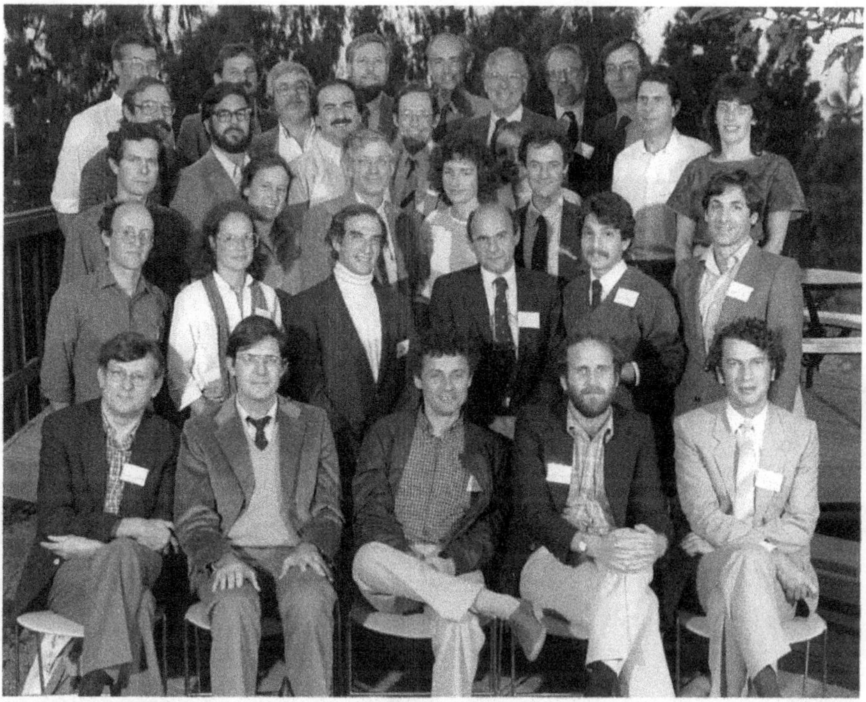

Figure 3: Symposium on learning and memory at UCI circa 1985. The symposium gathered a number of leaders in the field of learning and memory. Gary Lynch is seating in the middle of the first row and I am seating on the right of the first raw. Richard Morris is on the left of the third row behind Lynn Nadel (2nd row). Jim McGaugh, the director of the CNLM, is the fifth from the left on the 5th row. Richard Granger is standing behind me on my right.

Richard Morris had just invented a novel learning task, which now is associated with his name, the so-called Richard Morris water maze (Fig. 4). In this task, the rat or the mouse has to swim in a milky swimming pool until it finds a submerged platform allowing it to rest; the rat uses visual cues in the room to learn the location of the platform, since it is invisible for the rat. During this pivotal visit, I convinced Richard Morris to test the effects of a blocker of the NMDA receptors, referred to APV, in rats learning the water maze task (Fig. 4).

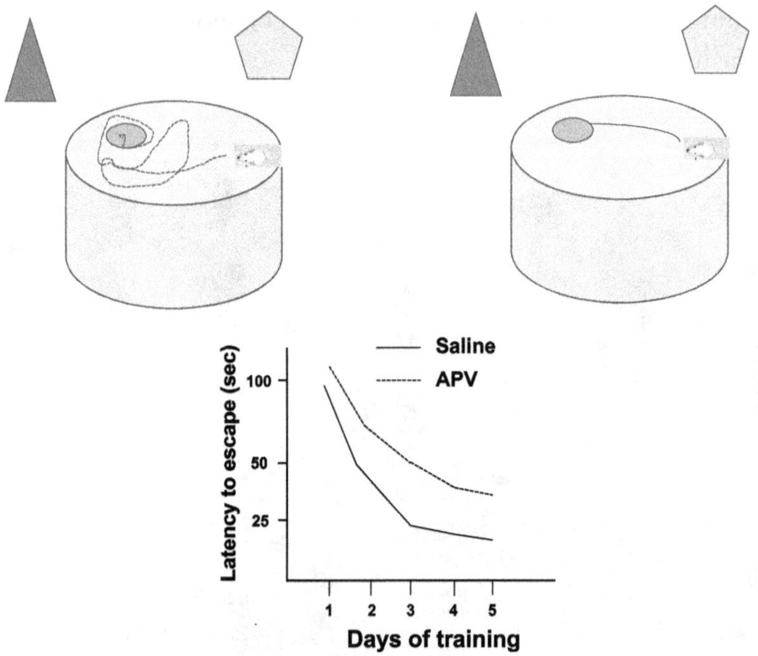

Figure 4: The Morris Water Maze: critical role of the NMDA receptor for learning and memory.

In this task, rats (or mice) are placed in a water pool rendered opaque by the addition of milk. They are swimming around until they find a hidden platform where they can rest. With successive training, rats learn the location of the platform by using visual cues located in the room. This results in a decrease in the time needed to find the platform (latency to escape). When rats were treated with the antagonist of the NMDA receptor, APV, they were significantly impaired in this task, as shown by the increase in latency to escape.

The experiment clearly showed that when APV was administered to the rat, the rat had difficulties learning the location of the submerged platform, while it was perfectly able to learn the location of a visible platform, indicating that the drug did not have any effect on swimming or on the animal's ability to perform a task in the swimming pool. Furthermore, Richard verified that APV injection was also able to block the induction of LTP in the hippocampus in live rats. The results were the first demonstration that the NMDA receptors were critically involved in this type of learning, which scientists classify as truly episodic learning, since the rat needs to associate the location of the platform with visual cues on the wall of the room (it is the similar type of learning we use to remember when we park our car in a parking structure, as we use a number of visual cues to do this). Our 1986 publication of the results in the prestigious Nature journal was widely acclaimed as a major breakthrough in our understanding of the mechanisms underlying learning and memory[8]. This finding had another important correlation, since the NMDA receptor is also a calcium channel, meaning that when activated, it leads to an influx of calcium in the dendritic spine. This was therefore the source of calcium that was needed to activate calpain and brought us back to the calpain hypothesis.

Confident that we had this task to help us understand the molecular mechanisms of learning and memory, I convinced Richard Morris to test the effects of a calpain inhibitor in this task. For this experiment, we decided to directly deliver a calpain inhibitor we had been using, leupeptin, in the rat brain ventricles, which provide an internal "irrigation" system for the brain. We started the treatment 2 days before training the animals and continued the treatment for the duration of the training (5 days). Surprisingly at that time, we did not find any effect of the inhibitor on learning[9]. This result contrasted with those we had obtained with the spatial maze and the olfactory discrimination tasks. However, several of the experimental conditions were very different. and in particular the training protocols were vastly different. For the spatial maze and the olfactory discrimination tasks, the training was very short, whereas for the Morris water maze, there were multiple trials each day and for several days. It took me almost 30 years to finally understand these paradoxical results.

As is so often the case in science, these early successes were quickly followed by major setbacks. The binding assay I was using to study glutamate receptors turned out to measure something completely different, throwing our whole published hypothesis for the mechanism of memory out of the window. It turned out that the assay I was using for analyzing binding of tritiated glutamate to its receptors, was not measuring binding to a receptor but was measuring its accumulation into vesicles formed from membrane fragments. We used several different ways to convince ourselves that this was indeed the case, and ultimately, we had to admit that we were not measuring glutamate binding to its receptors[10]. This was a major problem for our hypothesis since the increase in glutamate receptors we had proposed was a key step to explain the increase in synaptic strength. An increase in glutamate transport would have the opposite effect, as it would lead to a decrease in the number of glutamate molecules available to bind to its receptors. This was just another example illustrating how correct data (we knew the data were correct) can be misinterpreted leading to the wrong conclusions. This was also the first time this happened to me, and it really strongly affected me, the same way as some students used to always get As all of a sudden get a C. And as the saying says, "the higher you climb, the harder you fall." After our initial exhilaration came profound depression coupled with annoyance at the jubilation from competitors who did not hesitate to mock the UC Irvine work.

This was further exacerbated by the fact that the scientific community generally considered that a different calcium-dependent enzyme than calpain was involved in the formation of memory, which was a calcium-dependent protein kinase, calmodulin-dependent protein kinase[11]. This was difficult for us to understand for us, as protein kinases catalyze the reversible addition of a phosphate group to the side-chains of proteins, thereby only transiently modifying the functions of the proteins involved. These effects are transient since another class of enzymes, protein phosphatases, rapidly remove these phosphate groups. As we had argued, what was needed for a memory mechanism was a process that would lead to mostly irreversible modifications of some elements of the synapses, which made the calpain hypothesis so attractive since cleaving proteins is an irreversible process, as nobody has identified a mechanism that could "glue" back the cleaved pieces of a protein. Fortunately, resilience and persistence took over and stimulated me to turn the page and start over.

The hypothesis we had proposed contained too many elements that had the right features for a memory mechanism, making it very difficult to abandon it because some elements were wrong. As we discussed above, the calpain hypothesis was attractive because it provided a mechanism for a rapid and long-lasting modification of the structure of synaptic contacts, two features that were expected for a learning mechanism.

Because of this, I decided to keep working on the possible relationships between calpains and the glutamate receptors. Our rationale was that, if calpain was present in synaptic contacts and was activated by synaptic activity and cleaved cytoskeletal proteins, then it had to produce some long-lasting changes in synaptic contacts, which could be related to learning and memory.

One aspect that was particularly appealing was the fact that calpain activation resulted in the degradation of the protein spectrin, an essential element of the cell cytoskeleton. Neuronal communication is governed in part by the structural elements that define the shape of the cells and the shape of the synapses in neurons. Because shape regulates function, we were convinced that activation of calpain under conditions leading to changes in synaptic efficacy could indeed lead to structural alterations in synapses, which could lead to long-term memory formation. This idea was further supported by the fact that activation of NMDA receptors leads to an influx of calcium, the critical step in calpain activation. We therefore rewrote the initial hypothesis by focusing on this aspect, which emphasized the role of calpain activation on the regulation of the shape of dendritic spines, which could lead to more stable and stronger synapses[12]. Again, this hypothesis was supported by results from several laboratories, including Gary's lab, that LTP was associated with modifications of the shape of dendritic spines. This result was a heroic effort of a graduate student in Gary's lab with the help of two undergraduate students at UCI. Gary had an extraordinary talent to recruit undergraduate students and through the years, many of these students went on to have very successful academic career. In this case, the students spent days and weeks analyzing images taken with an electron microscope and measuring parameters related to the shape of synaptic contacts. The study was conducted blind, meaning that the students did not know if the images they were analyzing were from control slices or from slices that were exhibiting the LTP phenomenon. At the end, the data were decoded, and Gary and the students were amazed to find that after LTP, the synaptic contacts had changed their morphology from elliptical to spherical[13]. This result was also found in another lab and became an important element to further understand the mechanisms involved in synaptic plasticity and learning and memory.

Thus, despite the setback resulting from the fact that we were not labeling glutamate receptors in the binding assay, all the other results supported the notion that calpain was playing a significant role in synaptic plasticity and learning and memory. Many elements of the initial hypothesis were proven to be correct, as the NMDA receptors provided the influx of calcium needed for calpain activation, which would initiate a reorganization of the spine cytoskeleton and shape, and lead to a stronger and more stable synapse.

While I was happy at UCI, part of me was still missing Paris and my family and friends. I was told that there was an opportunity to become the head of a lab in a research institute in Paris dedicated to the study of aging. I did apply to the position of Director of Research at INSERM, and surprisingly I received notification that if I wanted to, I could get the job. I decided to go to Paris to take a closer look at the lab and the research institute. When I got there, I was completely shocked when the Director of the Institute showed me the lab I was supposed to move into. There were a bunch of monkey cages there and no lab at all! The Director tried to convince me that he would get the budget to build a real research lab. In addition, when I asked questions regarding the possibility of putting together a research team to work in the lab, I was told that I might be able to get a half-position for a technician plus the help of a Ph.D. student, who seemed lost in graduate school and whom nobody else wanted in their labs. Moreover, when I tried to negotiate with the INSERM the conditions for my return to France, I was told that I would not get any help at all. On top of that, I would have to take a significant cut in salary. Ultimately, I decided not to take the job and to stay at UCI. But this episode illustrates the difficulties that French scientists experience after they are strongly encouraged to go abroad for their postdoctoral training, while there is no real mechanism facilitating their return to France. I am told that the situation has changed now, but at the time, it was a significant issue.

Chapter 5
CALPAIN AND NEURODEGENERATION

While we were working on trying to understand the mechanisms underlying learning and memory, we needed to continue to investigate phenomena that Gary had discovered earlier and were funded by the NIH. In particular, the Lynch's lab had worked for several years on the question of what happened following denervation of a set of neurons receiving afferent projections from different inputs. In particular, the dentate gyrus in the hippocampus receives several types of inputs, including inputs from the entorhinal cortex and others from the commissural-association system. The granule cells project to a type of cell called polymorph neurons, which send projections back to the granule cells from both the ipsi-lateral (association) or contralateral (commissural) dentate gyrus. These projections are restricted to about 27% of the inner apical dendrites[1]. Since lesions of the entorhinal cortex were relatively easy to perform and result in the degeneration of the inputs from the entorhinal cortex to the dentate gyrus, the lab had studied what happened to the other inputs to the granule cells. Using a variety of techniques, Gary's lab had shown that this lesion resulted in the "sprouting" of the afferents of the commissural-association pathway (Fig. 1), meaning that these afferents were now expanding into the territory previously occupied by the inputs from the entorhinal cortex[1]. In fact, the discovery of the sprouting phenomenon was probably the first one that made Gary famous and got him interviews by TV and news channels, as it represented a clear demonstration that adult brains exhibited the ability to rewire themselves following some types of insults. It was therefore hoped that this rewiring mechanism could help a number of patients to recover from brain injuries. As it turned out, even some 40 years later, this finding has not led to significant advance in the management of these patients.

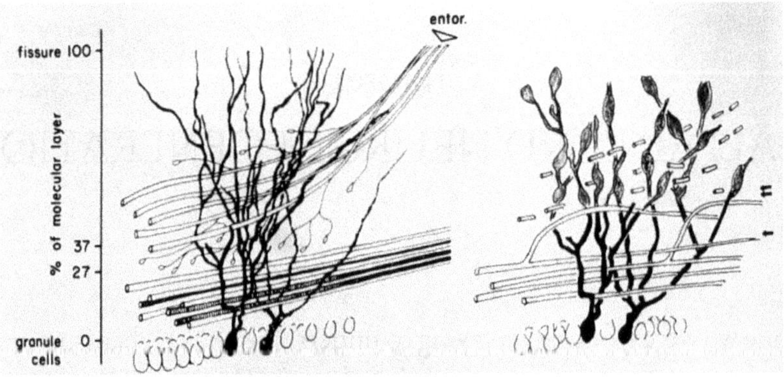

Figure 1: Illustration of sprouting after lesion. The entorhinal cortex sends axons that make synapses to the dendrites of the granule cells of the dentate gyrus (left). Following lesion of the entorhinal cortex, these axons degenerate (right). The axons from the other inputs to the granule cells expand in the denervated territories and make contacts to the dendrites (double arrows). (From Lynch and Baudry, 1983[1])

As these experiments were continuously going on, we decided to investigate whether calpain activation could be involved in the rewiring process. These studies led us to realize that calpain activation could under certain conditions result in neurodegeneration. In this case, the notion was that prolonged activation of calpain could lead to irreversible changes in cell function, resulting in the activation of death pathways. We found that calpain was activated in the degenerating neurons and the time-course of activation did match the time-course of degeneration, supporting the idea that calpain activation was causally involved in the degeneration process. Calpain was activated as early as 4 h after the lesion, was maximally activated at 2 days and remained activated for at least 27 days[2]. In this study, we used an assay that measured a fragment of spectrin generated by calpain-mediated cleavage as a marker for calpain activation. This assay has since then become a standard assay for analyzing calpain activation, as it can be used by biochemical analysis as well as by immunohistochemistry, which allows the visualization of this fragment in the brain (Fig. 2).

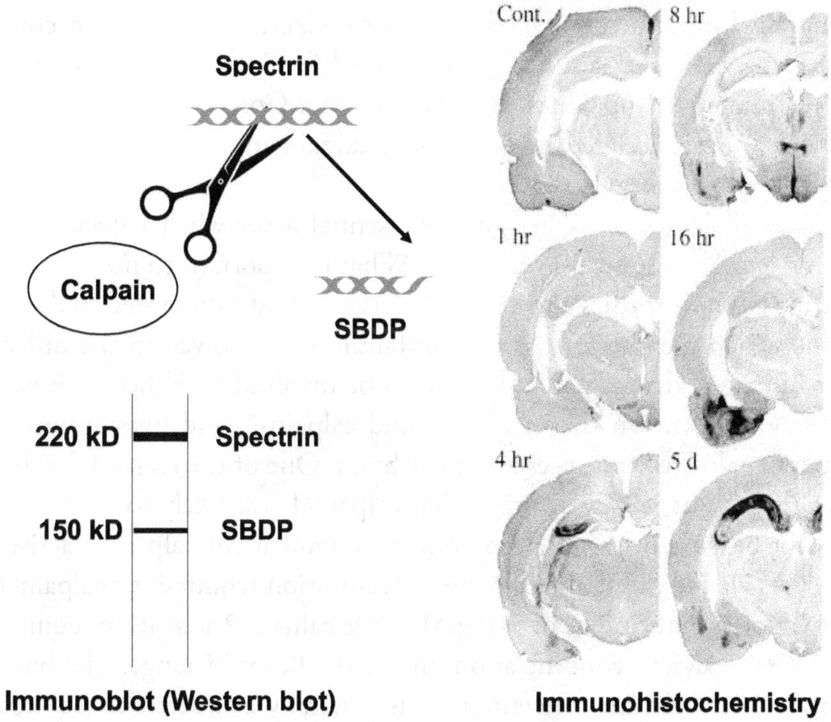

Figure 2: Standard assay for calpain activity.

This assay takes advantage of the fact that activated calpain cleaves the cytoskeletal spectrin to produce a spectrin breakdown product (SBDP). SBDP can be analyzed by using a western blot (a method to separate proteins based on their size/molecular weight) and labeling them with an antibody against spectrin, which recognizes both the native protein (molecular weight of 220 kD) and the fragment (molecular weight 150 kD). Alternatively, SBDP can be analyzed by immunohistochemistry (a method to label proteins in fixed brain sections) using an antibody specifically recognizing SBDP. In the example, brain sections were taken from mouse brains at various times after seizure activity elicited by the administration of a neurotoxin, kainic acid[3].

This set of results led Gary Lynch together with some of his colleagues at UC Irvine, to start a biotech company, called Cortex Pharmaceuticals, with the idea that calpain inhibitors could protect against neurodegeneration. This was in 1986, and for many years, Cortex Pharmaceuticals did provide many results suggesting that calpain inhibitors could indeed be neuroprotective following ischemic damage, mimicking what happens in stroke patients. Ultimately, the calpain inhibitor program from Cortex was transferred to Alkermes, the Boston company my friend Bernard had worked in, while Cortex was focusing on developing the Ampakines. However, neither Cortex Pharmaceuticals or Alkermes succeeded in developing calpain inhibitors for treating neurodegenerative diseases.

Nevertheless, Cortex became an essential actor when I decided to start NeurAegis some 30 years later. What is important to note is that, during all these studies and even at Cortex, nobody attempted to determine which member of the calpain family was involved in the different functions that calpain appeared to be involved in, although it was already well known that calpain-1 and calpain-2, and possibly other types of calpains, were present in the brain. One of the reasons for this was that it was widely assumed that calpain-1 was likely to be critical variant because of the high calcium requirement for calpain-2 activation. As we indicated, the calcium concentration required for calpain-1 activation is in the range of 5-10 μM, while calpain-2 activation requires very high calcium concentration, in the 0.2-0.4 mM range. The basal intracellular calcium concentration is generally estimated to be 0.02 to 0.05 μM, while the extracellular calcium concentration is in the 1-3 mM range. Intracellular calcium concentration is maintained at these low concentrations by sequestration in various intracellular organelles, as well as by multiple pumps that specifically pump calcium out of the cells. As we discussed above, calcium can enter neurons following the activation of various receptor/channels, such as the NMDA receptors, or by release from intracellular calcium stores. Under these conditions, intracellular calcium concentration can rise 10-100-fold for very short periods of time. This could potentially be sufficient to briefly activate calpain-1 in some very selective subcellular compartments. But this made it difficult to understand how calpain-2 could be activated at all. Despite these difficulties, we already proposed a model that could account for the differential activation of calpain-1and calpain-2 (Fig. 3).

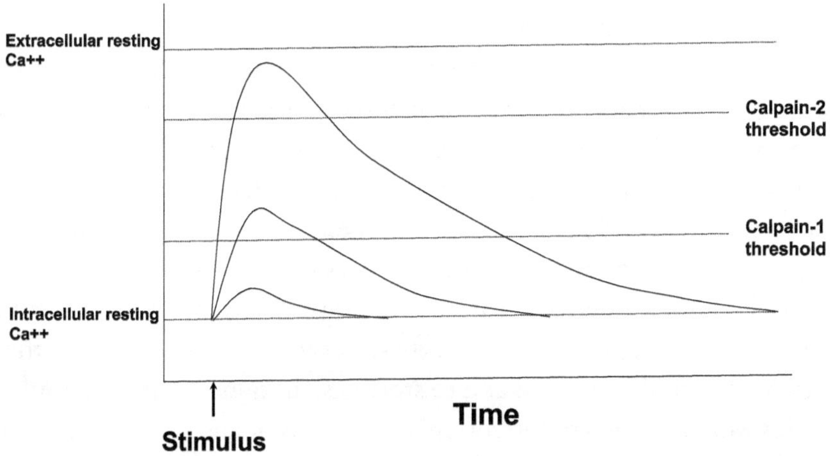

Figure 3: Schematic representation for the differential activation of calpain-1 and calpain-2.

Intracellular concentration of calcium is very low about 20-50 nM, whereas the extracellular concentration of calcium is about 2 mM. Many stimuli produced a brief and small increase in intracellular calcium concentration not sufficient to activate either calpain-1 or calpain-2. Some stimuli will produce an increase in calcium concentration sufficient to activate calpain-1, and this activation will rapidly terminate as calcium concentration decreases below the calpain-1 activation threshold. In rare cases, a stimulus will result in an increase in calcium concentration high enough to locally activate calpain-2. But this activation will also terminate, although additional mechanisms exist that will make this activation very long-lasting (discussed later). Modified from Lynch and Baudry[4].

Another reason for the lack of discussion regarding which member of the calpain family was involved in any study was the lack of selective inhibitors for the various members of the family. I, myself was as guilty as everybody else, as the question of which calpain isoform was involved in synaptic plasticity or neurodegeneration was really not a priority for me at the time. This would become the focus of later studies.

During this period, Gary connected with a computer scientist at UC Irvine, Richard Granger, and they became interested in the topic of neural networks, which started to be a hot topic in neuroscience. In particular, several physicists were interested in exploring the possibility of using artificial neural networks to perform computation. This was notably the case of Dr. Leon Cooper, who received the Nobel prize in physics for the BCS theory of superconductivity, and who was at Brown University where he founded the Institute for Brain and Neural Systems. Leon Cooper is also prominently featured in the George Johnson book mentioned earlier, as Leon Cooper was also interested in understanding how memories could be stored in neural networks[5]. But what Gary and Richard wanted to do was to work with neural networks with properties as close to those found in the brain as possible and incorporate rules of synaptic plasticity derived from the biology. When they implemented these rules of synaptic plasticity in these networks, they found that these networks were able to learn and to store vast amount of information[6].

This work attracted the attention of venture capitalists (VC) and in particular, that of Kevin Kinsella from Avalon Ventures in San Diego. Kevin knew a lot of people in the computer business in Silicon Valley and introduced Gary to Federico Faggin, the well-known Italian physicist, engineer, and the inventor of the first microprocessor, the Intel 4004. As Gary did not like to travel alone, he convinced Richard and me to join him during his visits to Silicon Valley to talk to Federico Faggin. We had numerous meetings with Federico and several computer scientists and tried to educate them on the architecture of the brain, the nature of synaptic transmission and the rules of synaptic plasticity. Conversely, they tried to educate us on the architecture of computers, the design and functions of chips, the functioning of transistors, and the building of large integrated circuits. The goals of these meetings were to evaluate the possibility of building new types of computers functioning more like the human brain than traditional computers. Retrospectively, it is clear that this idea was too premature, and we had a hard time finding a common language. Nevertheless, as discussed previously, Gary and Federico founded a company, which became Synaptics, and Carver Mead joined Federico to build different products based on pattern recognition. After a year or so of back-and-forth meetings, they thanked us for the ideas we had brought and concluded that they no longer needed us. Interestingly, Federico Faggin later returned to the study of brain networks when he founded in 2011 the "Federico and Elvia Foundation", which is dedicated to support the study of consciousness.

Gary has many interests besides the study of learning and memory, such as baseball, the Civil War, and historical Jesus. Another question that fascinated Gary Lynch was that of brain evolution, and he ended up writing a book on this topic "Big brain: the origins and future of brain intelligence"[7]. One particular aspect of this question, which he pursued was the relationship between brain size and lifespan across species. He spent hours collecting data from the literature and finally concluded that brain size was one of the best predictors of longevity, at least for mammals. However, one of the mammals he collected data for deviated from the relationship, and this was the bat, aka chyroptera. Bats have a much longer lifespan than their brain size predicts and the reason for this was never clearly understood. Because of the role of calpain in regulating cell shape, Gary and I started discussing the idea that maybe calpain was one of the factors contributing to brain size, and therefore to longevity. This was not too far-fetched, as brain size is related to the overall size of neuronal cells, which can be very long as some cells in the motor cortex extend all the way to the bottom of the spinal cord, and they are obviously very different in different types of mammals. I started collecting data on the levels of calpain activity in brains from all kinds of animals, ranging from birds to fish to horses. I ended up chasing opossum in the parking lot of UC Irvine at night. In the end, I succeeded in getting data for brain calpain activity in a fairly large number of species. It is important to note that at that time, we did not have the regulations we now have for the use of animals in experimental research. I am not sure I would be able to perform these studies now. For each of the brain we collected we measured calpain activity in various brain structures, but mostly in the cortex. We made some very interesting discoveries. First of all, calpain activity in the cortex was inversely related to brain size, meaning that large brains had less calpain activity than small brains (Fig. 4)[8]. Second, when we plotted brain calpain activity against lifespan, we did obtain a significant negative correlation, indicating indeed that calpain activity plays a significant role in determining the lifespan of a species, with species with long life expectancy having low levels of brain calpain activity. In fact, the slope of this relationship was – 1, which means that brain calpain activity in a given species is a very good predictor of its lifespan. Furthermore, we managed to get some bat brains because a colleague at UC Irvine was investigating the smell system in bats and one of his postdocs used to go to Napa and catch bats in church towers at night. Interestingly, bat brains had lower calpain activity than predicted by their body weight and furthermore, bat brain calpain activity was perfectly in line with their longevity compared to the other mammals (Fig. 4)[9].

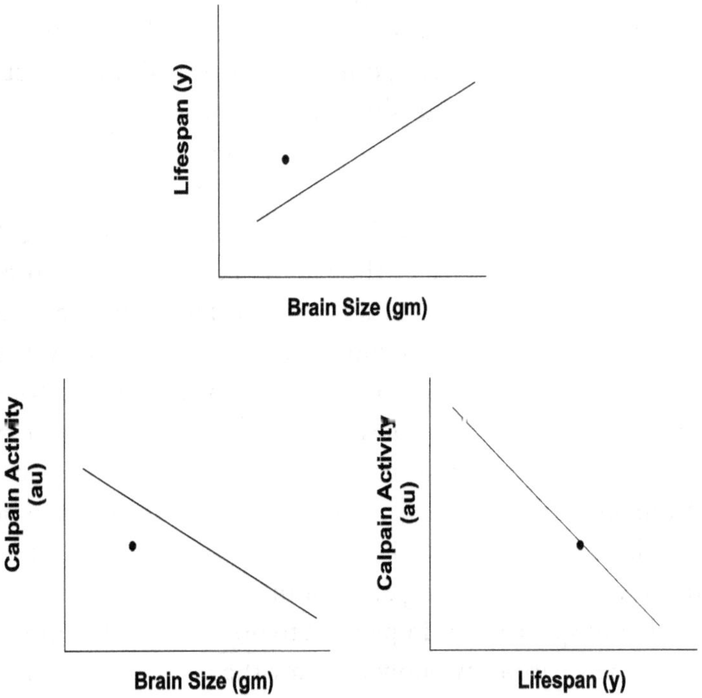

Figure 4. Relationship between calpain activity, brain size, and lifespan across mammalian species.

Top: Lifespan is positively correlated with brain size. Lower left: Calpain activity in cortex is negatively related to brain size. Lower right: Calpain activity is negatively correlated with lifespan and the slope of the relationship is -1. The dot represents the values for the bats, chyroptera. On the top and left charts, the values significantly deviate from the expected values for the brain size. However, on the lower right chart, the value fits perfectly with the predicted value.

Our interpretation from these strange results was that calpain activity was regulating the stability of neurons and therefore low levels of calpain activity in large neurons represented a neuroprotective function of calpain. The real explanation for these findings would become much clearer about 30 years later.

Looking back at this period of time, it is difficult to convey the feelings, the excitement, and the sense of accomplishment, but also the pain, the doubts, and the fear of failure. Despite having been fired by the CNRS, I had published 120 papers in 12 years, an average of 10 papers a year. I had submitted several grants and got funded by the National Science Foundation and the National Institute of Health, and I had climbed the academic ladder, moving up from postdoc to Assistant Professor and to Associate Professor, albeit in the in-residence category, as indicated previously. The UC system has a parallel system from the regular faculty position, which is called the in-residence program[10]. The system gives scientists a faculty position, as long as the faculty can provide his/her salary from external sources. While this is a good deal for the university, since it does not need to provide a salary while still having an additional faculty member who can serve on committees, train students and occasionally teach, it is much more stressful for the faculty, as he/she needs to continually apply for funding to cover the salary. I was on this system and, while I was repeatedly told that if a regular faculty position became available, I could apply for it, I knew that it was not likely to happen. But for the most part, I did not really care; I was working hard, I was spending a lot of time with my mentor, Gary Lynch, I was learning a lot about science and lots of other topics Gary was interested in, and the lab was an amazing incubator of ideas and opinions.

I remember vividly an episode when it had been raining for days (quite an unusual event for Southern California) and Campus security came to the lab and told us that we had to leave before the roads around the campus would become flooded. Everybody said, "We don't care, we are staying in the lab and will sleep here if necessary." I am not sure that this would be the reaction of lab personnel nowadays. The lab was very international, and there were quite a few French postdocs and students, a Japanese postdoc, three Swiss postdocs and for a brief period one German postdoc. It was not uncommon for all the French-speaking people from the lab to be talking in the hallway in French to the surprise of all the undergraduate students walking around. We also had many French dinners, and we even introduced the game of petanque on the

UCI Campus[11], as a few French postdocs were from the South of France where this game is mostly practiced.

UCI had built houses for faculty and staff around the campus, and I was living in one of these houses, which was nice, as I could just walk to the lab. Often, I would be walking and running into the famous physicist, Fred Reines. I remember him telling me that I should read the book "Nobel Dreams"[12], which relates the story regarding how another physicist, Carlo Rubia won his Nobel Prize. It was clear that Fred was dreaming himself about the Nobel Prize since he had discovered the neutrino, and his dream came true in 2015. However, by then his mental health had already started to decline and I am not sure he was able to enjoy his fame and glory for a significant amount of time.

It is also worth stressing that the calpain hypothesis of learning and memory was unique and very much ahead of its time; while the majority of scientists did not accept it at the time, it has since resisted the passage of time and can even be seen in some textbooks. Gary and I also had succeeded in contributing to the discovery that calpain participates not only in synaptic plasticity and learning and memory, but also in neuronal remodeling after lesions and in neurodegeneration. True, we did not solve the puzzle then, but we put some significant pieces on the board, maybe even enough to start seeing a glimpse of the final image.

In many ways, this is how science works, by little steps and rarely by giant leaps, although these do happen once in a blue moon. Gary also taught me not to be afraid of thinking big, of keeping my eyes on the big picture and trying to integrate all the information at hand into the largest framework as possible. He also taught me the necessity to confirm and to reconfirm every result using different approaches to make sure that each finding was solid and reproducible. This was also a remarkable lesson, and I have been trying to apply this principle ever since.

I kept hoping I would get a more secure position at UC Irvine, but the local political situation was not playing in my favor. In addition, as much as I enjoyed working with Gary Lynch, I knew that it was time for me to move on and to "fly on my own." This was going to be the next stage of my scientific career.

Chapter 6
MOVING FROM UCI TO USC

For personal reasons, in the Fall of 1988, I took a sabbatical year to go work at Genentech in South San Francisco as a visiting scientist. At that time, Genentech was still relatively small, but it was still an impressive campus, with a truly academic orientation. Everybody was cloning, and I, of course, attempted to clone calpains. This type of experiment was indeed quite different from what I had been doing until this point. It required me to be very careful and rigorous, and I had a lot of trouble to manage this technology. It took me my whole year at Genentech to manage to obtain a few clones, which I brought back with me when I left Genentech to go back to UCI in June 1989. I also started running regularly, inspired by the encouragement of the French friend I mentioned previously and with whom I reconnected with at Genentech, Bernard Malfroy, who would become a key figure in the quest to find a drug to treat concussion. Bernard was a dedicated marathon runner, and at some point, he was running one marathon a month. He also ended up writing a book "Marathoning through life"[1] in which he relates two parallel stories, his quest to run the Boston marathon, and his quest to find a treatment for a terrible disease, ataxia telengiectasia[2]. In particular, during this period, I ran with him the Napa Valley marathon, which was a wonderful experience, as one gets the opportunity to see many wineries along the roads and to dream of all the good wines they are producing.

Working at Genentech was a sharp contrast from working at UC Irvine. The working schedule was much more like 8:00am-5:00pm, and rarely did people work during the weekend. I did not have long discussions with people like Gary Lynch, since, as a visiting scientist, I was not implicated in any teams. I was working mostly in Bernard's lab, which I managed to contaminate with radioactive phosphorus, and this really annoyed his technician. Instead, I tried to enjoy life in San Francisco; however, coming from Los Angeles, I was surprised that San Francisco was actually pretty small, overcrowded and not easy to live in. I did some collaborative work with a scientist I had known as a postdoc at UCI, Dr. Tony Altar. Tony had a great sense of humor, and he made this comment when he was analyzing some data during the famous San Francisco earthquake of 1989: "my data are earthshaking but not to this extent!."

I still had my lab at UC Irvine during this period with a few people continuing to work there and I needed to spend some time talking to them and making sure the work was progressing. Another major difference between working in a company and working at the university is the distribution of resources. At Genentech, there were rooms filled with pieces of equipment, most of them still wrapped in their original cases and boxes. On the other hand, there were no undergraduate students who could help running experiments and very limited technical support. All the scientists had to do pretty much everything themselves. This is where I realized that I was not particularly good at running experiments by myself, and that I needed a team of people around me to run experiments.

During this period, I was contacted by Professor Richard Thompson who had been recruited by the University of Southern California (USC) in Los Angeles from Stanford, where he moved while I was still at UCI. Under the direction of a physicist, Dr. Bill Wagner, and a neurobiologist, Dr. Bill McClure, USC had a very ambitious plan to become the world leader in neurosciences. As discussed earlier, I had known Richard when he was at UC Irvine and with whom I had collaborated and whom I highly respected. He was charged by USC to recruit a multidisciplinary team of scientists to form the Center for Neural, Informational and Behavioral Sciences (NIBS) and to fill up a new neuroscience building on the University Park Campus, the Hedco Neuroscience Building (Fig. 1). This was a very smart move from USC, as USC had a very strong School of Engineering, with an outstanding group of computer scientists. Thus, the idea of bringing together psychologists, neurobiologists, and computer scientists was very timely and judicious.

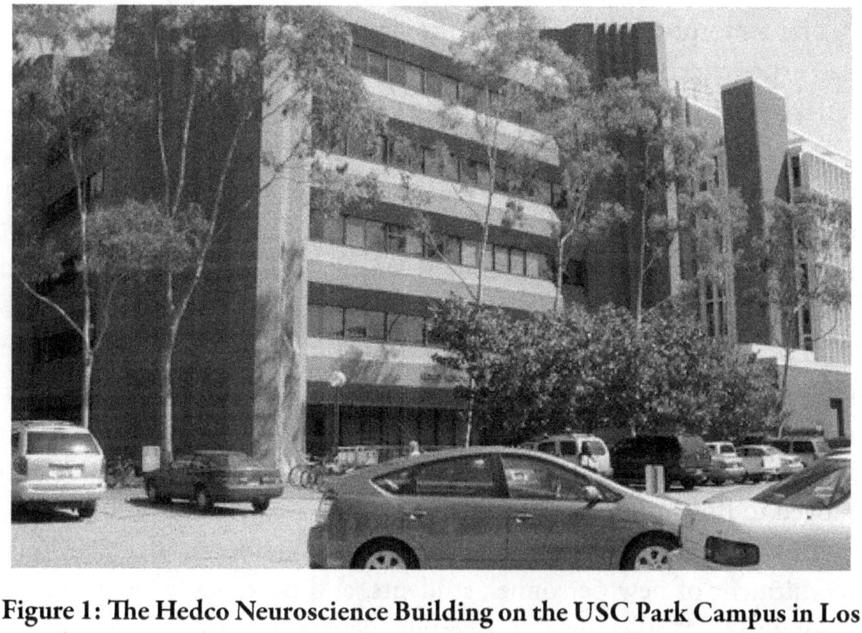

Figure 1: The Hedco Neuroscience Building on the USC Park Campus in Los Angeles.

My laboratory was located on the third floor and I spent 23 years there.

In fact, a few years before, Bill Wagner had tried to recruit Gary Lynch to move to USC to head the multidisciplinary institute he wanted to start at USC. I remember him and Bill McClure coming to Irvine and having lunch with Gary and me, as they were trying to convince Gary to move to LA. Ultimately, Gary declined the offer and Drs. Wagner and McClure went on to recruit Richard Thompson as the Director of NIBS. Richard really wanted me to join NIBS and to bring my expertise in biochemistry to complement the computational scientists, anatomists and behavior scientists he had already recruited. This was quite exciting, and on top of that, I would have a regular faculty position and my own laboratory space in the new Hedco Building. I did try to get a counter-offer from UC Irvine, but the leadership was not interested in keeping me there, and I accepted the position at USC. In September 1989, after my year at Genentech, I moved my lab from UCI to USC, in the neurobiology section of the department of biological sciences in the Hedco Neuroscience building. This was an exciting time again, which is always the case when one moves to a new position and a new lab.

The atmosphere at USC was also completely different from what I had experienced at UCI. Everybody wanted to collaborate, and my lab quickly got involved in many projects with other scientists in the neuroscience section of the Department of Biology, in the School of Gerontology where there were several neuroscientists, as well as in the neurology department at USC Medical School. Richard Thompson, a member of the American National Academy of Sciences, and a leader in the field of learning and memory, had, like he did at UCI, a very dynamic lab with many postdocs and graduate students, and he became my second mentor. He had a French postdoc in his lab, Dr. Georges Tocco, and we rapidly became friends. Georges contributed enormously to the experiments my lab was performing. He was later recruited by Eukarion and moved to Boston.

The advantage of doing research in universities is the continual recruitment of new personnel, students, and postdocs, to work in the laboratories. While there is a certain degree of chance in recruiting good students and postdocs, the process does work and is the engine of progress and the necessary component for preparing the next generation of scientists. When I started at USC, I had brought with me from UCI a postdoctoral fellow from Lebanon, Dr. Imad Najm, and I also recruited a new postdoc from Canada, Dr. Guy Massicotte. Imad left after a few years to take a position at the Cleveland Clinic where he is now the Director of the Epilepsy Program. Guy came from the University of Trois-Rivieres in Quebec and was a great scientist and a great person. I ended up visiting him back in Trois-Rivieres where he got a faculty position after he left my lab. He really made me appreciate the unique features of Quebec and of the Quebecois language. I also quickly recruited a graduate student from the new NIBS graduate program. The lab was small, and we were all working at the bench trying to establish the lab as quickly as possible. Guy Massicotte eagerly began working on an alternative hypothesis to explain synaptic plasticity, implicating a different calcium-dependent enzyme, phospholipase A2. This enzyme is also a degradative enzyme, but instead of cleaving proteins like proteases do, it cleaves phospholipids, which are the main constituent of membranes. While the idea was attractive, it was difficult to integrate it in the framework that I had developed over the previous 10 years. But I agreed to let him work on his idea since it was a calcium-dependent enzyme and its activation also resulted in long-lasting modifications of cell structure and properties. In particular, we showed that its activation resulted in alterations of the properties of glutamate receptors[3], which remained a central element of the working hypothesis Gary and I had proposed 10 years earlier. We developed new assays for studying these receptors and recruited an army of undergraduate students to help with the experiments. USC was certainly a great place for this, as Los Angeles is clearly an attractive city for national and international students.

Shortly after I started at USC, I was surprised to see a large number of students dragging a little bear in the dirt on the USC campus. Intrigued, I asked some of my students the meaning of such a behavior. Again, they looked at me as if I was coming from another planet and told me it was because of the "Big Game", meaning the annual football game between USC and its rival from across town, UCLA. Thus, the USC students protected their beloved statue of a Trojan standing in front of the Administration building, and were demeaning the mascot of UCLA, a little bruin. I have to admit that although I spent 23 years at USC, I only went to the Coliseum to watch the USC Trojans play football only twice. Shame on me, I guess!

During this period, I also got involved in another biotech company with my friend Bernard Malfroy, who started Eukarion, Inc, a biotech focusing on developing novel antioxidant molecules, which were mimics of natural enzymes playing such a role in living tissues, namely superoxide oxidase (SOD) and catalase. Bernard had left Genentech at the same time I moved to USC, as he had been recruited by a new biotech company in Boston, Alkermes. He worked there for a few years before he felt he needed to start his own company. He asked me to join him in this adventure, which was based on his finding an interesting molecule discovered by a scientist at Duke University, desferrioxamine-manganese, which exhibited SOD activity[4]. Bernard did not hesitate to go to Duke University and to negotiate a licensing agreement for the use of this molecule in exchange for some equity in Eukarion. My lab at USC became for a while Eukarion's lab, and Bernard spent quite some time traveling from Boston to Los Angeles to run experiments. By serendipity, a year later, Bernard identified a new family of molecules, which he thought could be potential SOD mimetics. He named these molecules EUK-n, and several of these molecules were synthesized and tested over the years, starting with what he called EUK-8. We did test them and found they were indeed very potent SOD-catalase mimetics (Fig. 2)[5], and we used them in many animal models of diseases in which excess free radical formation was postulated to be involved (see Chapter 8). We had great success in the lab, but that did not translate in either business success or clinical applications. While Bernard was able to raise funding and to run Eukarion for several years, we did not succeed in bringing one of these molecules to the clinic. One of the major findings we made, which again was taken up by the popular press (a cartoon in the Boston Globe) was that giving one of these molecules to the roundworm Caenorhabditis Elegans, generally called C. Elegans, greatly extended its lifespan[6].

This finding provided clear evidence that excess free radicals contribute to the aging process and that it could be possible to extend lifespan by finding ways to eliminate excess free radical formation. In any event, one of these molecules, EUK-134, made it to the cosmetic field and is still present in some anti-aging creams, as discussed in Chapter 1. As Bernard put it, how many biotech companies can claim to bring one of their products to the marketplace. This was my first attempt at being a co-founder in a biotech company and taught me a few valuable lessons.

In our continued quest to find potential calcium-dependent mechanisms that could regulate glutamate receptors, we got a remarkable result, which happens once in a while in science. It was an effect so black and white that we could see it with the naked eye, which is quite rare in biology, as most of the time one needs some sophisticated equipment to observe the results of experiments (Fig. 3). In this case, we clearly

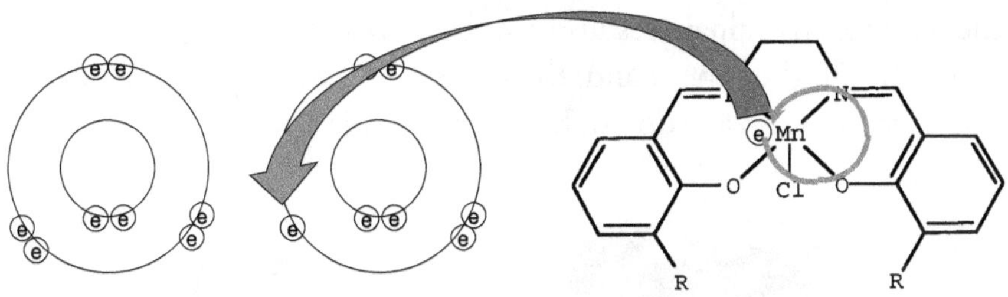

Oxygen (O_2)   Oxygen Free Radical ($O_2^{\bullet -}$)

EUK-8: R = H
EUK-134: R = OCH_3

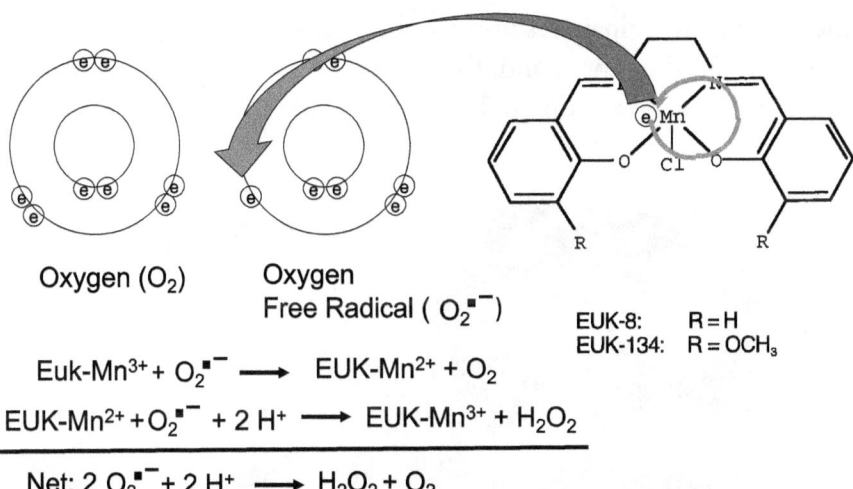

$$\text{Euk-Mn}^{3+} + O_2^{\bullet -} \longrightarrow \text{EUK-Mn}^{2+} + O_2$$

$$\text{EUK-Mn}^{2+} + O_2^{\bullet -} + 2\,H^+ \longrightarrow \text{EUK-Mn}^{3+} + H_2O_2$$

$$\text{Net: } 2\,O_2^{\bullet -} + 2\,H^+ \longrightarrow H_2O_2 + O_2$$

Figure 2: EUKns are potent SOD mimetics.

The molecule of oxygen (top left) has 4 pairs of electrons. The loss of one electron results in the formation of the oxygen free radical. On the right is the structure of two of the EUKn molecules, EUK-8 when R is hydrogen and EUK-134 when R is a methoxy group (OCH_3). Because the manganese in EUKn can cycle between Mn+++ and Mn++, it can donate one electron to the oxygen free radical, restoring the oxygen molecule. The overall reaction is exactly what the enzyme superoxide dismutase (SOD) is doing, justifying the definition of the EUKn molecules as SOD-mimetics.

demonstrated that calpain activation resulted in the truncation of one subtype of the glutamate receptors, the AMPA receptors. We were using tissue sections, which we incubated without or with calcium, and then we would label the receptors with an antibody to the receptors to visualize the location and levels of receptors in different brain regions. Adding calcium to the incubation dramatically altered the distribution of the receptors. They were gone from many regions and surprisingly appeared in other regions. This effect was almost completely blocked with a calpain inhibitor. As can be seen in the figure, which one can see with the naked eye, is that the receptors disappear from the dendritic fields in the hippocampus, and also from most of the cortical regions. Surprisingly, it seems that the staining gets darker in the cell bodies of the hippocampal neurons. The decrease in staining is best explained by the truncation of the receptors by calpain resulting in the loss of immunoreactivity of the antibody. On the other hand, the increase in staining is quite puzzling and to this day, I really do not have a clear explanation.

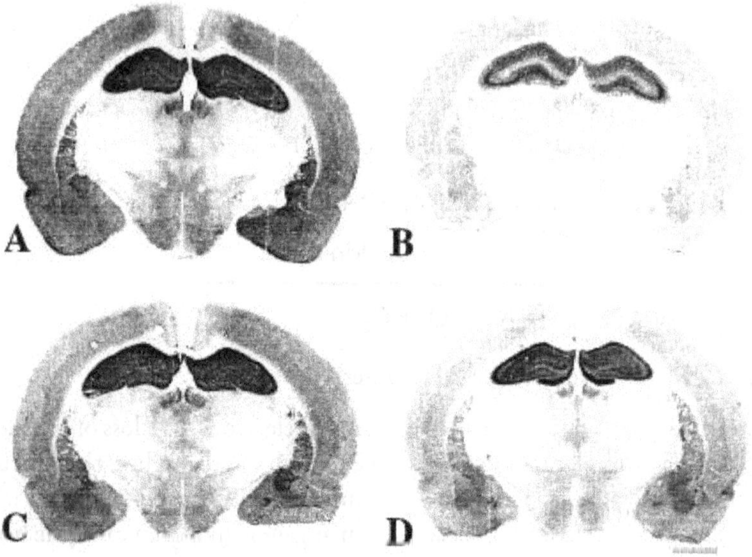

Figure 3: Effects of calcium on AMPA glutamate receptors.

Fresh frozen rat brain sections were incubated in the absence (A,C) or presence (B-D) of calcium for 30 min, and without (A,B) or with (C,D) a calpain inhibitor. After that they were processed for immunohistochemistry with antibodies against the AMPA glutamate receptors. As can readily be seen, calcium treatment dramatically reduced the staining. The presence of the calpain inhibitor almost completely prevented the decrease in staining[7]. (Figure 1 from Bi et al., Neuroreport. 6: 61-64, 1994, reproduced with permission).

While this did not provide a clear link to our original hypothesis, it did indicate that calpain was involved in the regulation of glutamate receptors and therefore of synaptic transmission at the synapses using glutamate as a neurotransmitter. These results provided clear evidence that at least part of our original hypothesis was true, and we frenetically worked to revise it to account for the new findings. We then exerted considerable effort to identify other proteins that could be cleaved by calpain and participate in the regulation of synaptic plasticity. And yes, we found a whole bunch of them! Thus, we identified that calpain could also cleave another subtype of glutamate receptors, the NMDA receptors[8], as well as several synaptic proteins involved in anchoring the receptors to the synaptic membranes[9]. At that time, it was still relatively easy to publish new findings in the scientific literature, something that has changed drastically since. This provided a great reward mechanism for students and postdocs and for their completion of Ph.D. and for their future careers, respectively. It was also a great tool to disseminate our findings to the scientific community and to get invited to meetings and conferences.

It was also a valuable metric for grant evaluators to determine the productivity of laboratories and the allocation of research funding to principal investigators. During this period, I succeeded in getting funding from both the National Science Foundation and from the National Institute of Health to support my research activities. As we shall see later, the situation has changed significantly in recent years. At that time, it seemed that if you were working hard, published good manuscripts, trained graduate students and postdocs, the chances of getting your work funded were relatively high; approximately 30% of the submitted applications were getting funded. This number has now decreased to below 10% for many Institutes of the National Institutes of Health, making the process much more difficult.

In the late 1990s, I received a phone call from a very distinguished French neuroscientist, Dr. Ladislav Tauc, who had a very famous laboratory just outside of Paris. Dr. Tauc is also famous because he trained another famous neuroscientist and Nobel Laureate, Dr. Eric Kandel, who started his work using the sea slug Aplysia to understand the mechanisms of learning and memory[10] in the laboratory of Dr. Tauc. Dr. Tauc explained to me that he was planning to retire and asked me if I would be interested in taking over his laboratory at Gif sur Yvette, outside of Paris. I told him I was very flattered that he would consider me as his successor and told him I would think about it. This sounded like a very attractive opportunity, and I decided to call a few friends in Paris to ask their opinion. They were all unanimous to tell me that this was a politically very charged situation and that there were lots of people who were eager to take over the lab; if I would decide to come, they would make my life very miserable. They all concluded that I was much better off staying in the US, considering that the funding for research in France was nowhere comparable to the situation in the US. Moreover, after all the years I had spent in the US, I would have a very hard time to deal with the French system. Thus, I replied to Dr. Tauc that although I was very happy that he would consider me for his position, I had decided to stay at USC. This would be my last attempt to move back to France.

Even after moving to USC, I remained close to Gary Lynch, and we had many discussions regarding the fate of our original hypothesis and the difficulties we had to convince the scientific establishment of its value. In 2001, almost 20 years after we formulated the calpain hypothesis of learning and memory, we got an opportunity to review all the recent findings and to attempt to integrate them in a comprehensive review[11]. This was one of these moments all scientists dream of, as writing this review made us look back at what we did over the previous 20 years, and to see how the field had evolved, which was mostly by taking many turns, many steps backwards as well as forward. It was also the time to reminisce about the roles various people in our labs and in the scientific community had played during this period. Interestingly, in our review, we introduced the notion of silent synapses, defined as synapses lacking one of the subtypes of glutamate receptors responsible for the basic operation of these synapses, the AMPA receptors, which would therefore remain non-functional until some events would allow them to become active. Remember that the NMDA receptors require postsynaptic depolarization to be activated; in the absence of AMPA receptors, even if glutamate is released from the presynaptic terminal, there would not be sufficient depolarization to activate the NMDA receptors, and therefore there would not be a postsynaptic response, justifying the name of silent synapse. (Fig. 4).

We also postulated that calpain activation could be involved in unsilencing these synapses, which could provide a mechanism for learning. The existence of such synapses was demonstrated shortly after the review was published but nobody gave us credit for the idea, as is often the case in science. Nevertheless, writing this review reinforced our thinking that we had been on the right track since the beginning, and that all the elements of the complex puzzle were starting to fall into places. In some ways, we felt like mathematicians must feel when they demonstrate a

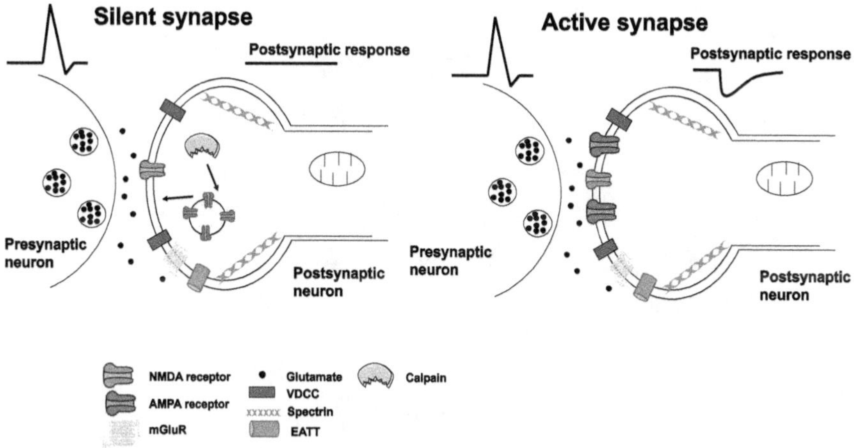

Figure 4: Unsilencing silent synapses.

On the left, a silent synapse has NMDA receptors but no AMPA receptors. When an action potential reaches the synaptic terminal, released glutamate does not elicit a postsynaptic response. On the left, unsilencing results in the insertion of AMPA receptors in the postsynaptic membrane and an action potential now elicits a postsynaptic response. Calpain activation might participate in the unsilencing.

theorem that had plagued the community for a long time. With retrospect, it is easy to see how difficult it is to convince the scientific community that one has solved a difficult problem, as there are always details that are going to be missing and critics will focus on these details. Gary and I loved to look at the big picture and were not too concerned about the millions of little details that remained unexplained.

During this period, a team of USC neuroscientists got involved in a research project funded by the pharmaceutical branch of the Japanese company, Suntory. Suntory is famous in the US for its whisky, and I had the opportunity to visit the company in Japan to review the progress of the research project. I was particularly impressed when some of the directors of Suntory took us to dinner in a restaurant and at the end of the dinner, they simply gave their business cards to the waiter who had brought the check. I had clearly never seen this done any place else. The pharmaceutical branch of Suntory ended up merging with Sankyo Pharmaceuticals and we continued our sponsored research for several years. I even had one of their scientists spend some time in my laboratory.

Chapter 7
BACK TO UCI

The scientific process is not linear and is not a continuous march forward. Instead, failures follow successes and negative results are as common as positive results. Since negative results are rarely published, this means that there are periods of time when a laboratory does not have new positive results to report. While our lab had published an average of 9 publications per year from 1988 to 2001, the pace of work slowed down in the lab at USC after that. I decided to take a sabbatical year from USC and to return to work at UCI with Gary Lynch. A sabbatical year means that a faculty member can take 6-12 months off from his/her current position and spend this time learning new skills, initiate new collaborations or explore new opportunities. This is another benefit of working in a university, as it is widely recognized that faculty members periodically need to "rejuvenate" and expand their horizons. In general, a faculty member can take one sabbatical year every 6-7 years. In addition, the university generally agrees to pay the faculty member 100% of the salary for 6 months, or 50% of the salary for 12 months.

By 2001 Gary's lab had moved across the UCI Campus to what was called the University Research Park, and quite interestingly, the address of the lab was 101 Theory. The Research Park had been created in 1996 to facilitate the spin-offs of companies created as a result of discoveries made by UCI scientists as well as to attract innovative companies by offering them access to UCI resources. This address became the title of a book written by a journalist from the *LA Times*, Terry McDermot, who like Georges Johnson had done before, spent a lot of time in Gary's lab to learn more about Gary's research and personality. He did write several articles for the *LA Times* and ultimately a book entitled "101 Theory: A neuroscientist's quest for memory"[1]. The book is an exciting description of what was going on in Gary's lab and is somewhat a follow-up from George Johnson's book. While George Johnson was a scientific writer, Terry McDermot was an investigative journalist, and his writing reflects his detailed analysis of the atmosphere and daily activities going on in Gary's lab. He and Gary became good friends, as they shared a lot of similar interests. By a strange twist of fame, it turns out that Terry McDermot lived in Manhattan Beach just across the street from one of my colleagues and friends at USC. Small World indeed!

Gary Lynch had started two new companies, Thorus Pharmaceuticals (Thorus) and Tensor Pharmaceuticals (Tensor), and this was the reason he moved his lab from the UCI Campus to the Research Park. When I discussed with Gary the idea of taking a sabbatical year from USC, he asked me to serve as Tensor VP Research. Tensor was developing a novel technology based on a multielectrode array, which allowed to stimulate and record multiple networks simultaneously and for several weeks, when using cultured hippocampal slices[2]. This was particularly interesting for such cultured slices, as we knew that hippocampal networks played a critical role in learning and memory (Fig. 1).

The general idea for Tensor was to develop the technology to the point that drugs acting on the nervous system could be categorized based on the pattern of effects they could elicit in this complex neuronal network. This Brain-on-Chip technology would become a tool for drug discovery.

In parallel, Thorus Pharmaceuticals was developing software for the analysis of EEG recorded from a scalp multielectrode array (Fig. 2), which could identify what type of neurological/neuropsychiatric disorders patients would present in order to provide the best treatment. In some aspect, Thorus was a complement of Tensor technology as well as a

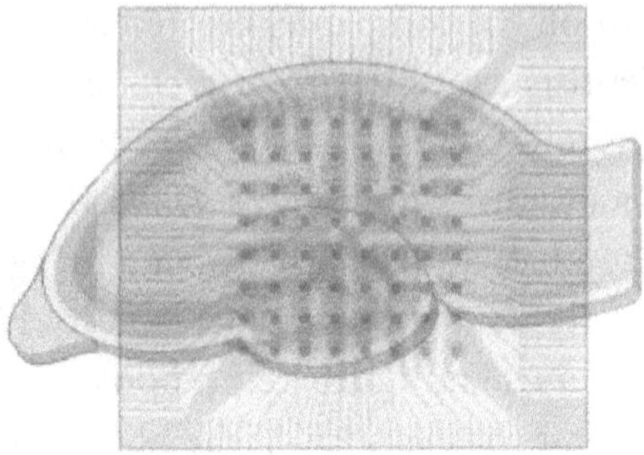

Figure 1: Multielectrode recording from a hippocampal slice.

A hippocampal slice is set on a multielectrode array. Stimulating and recording can be performed from any of the electrodes in the array, providing information regarding neuronal activity in the whole hippocampal circuitry.

precursor of what is now called personalized medicine. It is quite amazing that Thorus and Gary were again way ahead of the time, as Psychogenics, a well-known drug discovery company just launched what they call the eCube®, an Artificial-Intelligence (AI)-based pharmaco EEG platform to support drug discovery[3].

In addition, Gary was still very much involved in Cortex Pharmaceuticals, which was no longer developing calpain inhibitors but was now focusing on the development of a new class of molecules called positive AMPA receptor modulators or ampakines for the treatment of various indications. Gary asked me to also help with developing the ampakine program for Cortex.

Thus, in 2001, I was involved again with two of Gary's companies, Tensor and Cortex. Cortex at that time had a collaborative partnership with a French pharmaceutical company, Les Laboratoires Servier (www.servier.com), and I ended up going to Paris a few times for meetings with the Servier scientists. Tensor was funded by a grant from the State of California, and we were trying to get some investors interested in expanding its funding, although we knew that the company was still at an early stage.

While it was great to be back at UC Irvine and to work with Gary, all these activities did not allow me to spend much time to perform experiments directed at providing further evidence to support our original

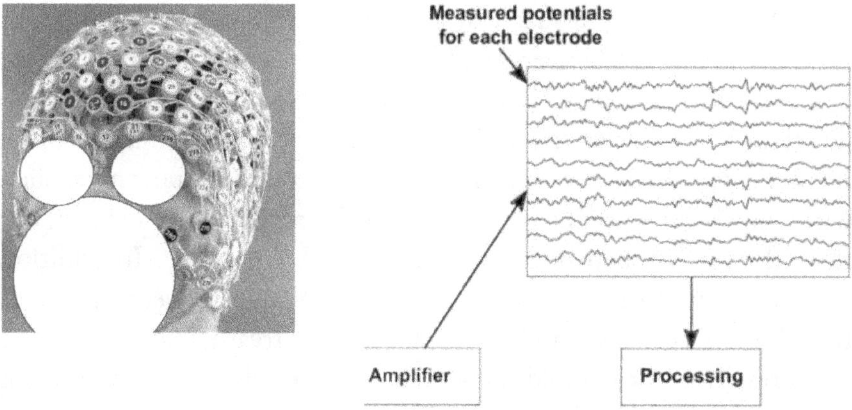

Figure 2: Human EEG recording from a multielectrode array.

A net with a large number of electrodes is set on the surface of the skull. Signals from all the electrodes are amplified and analyzed by special software to categorize various brain disorders.

hypothesis regarding the role of calpain in learning and memory or in neurodegeneration. Nevertheless, after my one year of sabbatical, I decided to stay one more year at UCI and took a one-year leave of absence from USC.

Another reason to stay one more year at UCI was my marriage to an amazing woman and scientist, Dr. Xiaoning Bi, who was working with Gary Lynch, and who became an essential component of all my future work on calpain. She had been my Ph.D. student at USC, and I had been extremely impressed by her intelligence, her kindness and her dedication to science. After graduating from USC, she started a post-doctoral period in Gary's lab and rapidly moved on to become an Assistant Professor in the Psychiatry Department at UCI. After reconnecting with her, we realized that we were a perfect match and decided to get married. She became my confidant, my collaborator, my inspiration, and my motivation to pursue work on calpain, although at times, she would make fun of me, saying "nobody cares about your calpain." She had developed her own research program and became interested in the role lysosomes play in neuronal function and dysfunction. Interestingly, she was recruited a few years later by a small private university in Southern California, Western University of Health Sciences located in Pomona.

During this period at UCI, I still managed to run some experiments directed at further understanding the functions of calpain in the brain. In particular, we discovered that treating cultured hippocampal slices with ampakines surprisingly resulted in the activation of calpain, and this effect was independent of the NMDA receptors[4]. In addition, such activation was not associated with any sign of neurodegeneration. Moreover, Gary's lab had also found that treating rats with ampakines resulted in the rapid increase in brain levels of a growth factor, brain-derived growth factor (BDNF)[5], which was known to play a very important role in neuronal growth and survival[6]. At the time, we did not understand the link between these 2 events triggered by the ampakines, calpain activation and increase in BDNF, and it took us several years to find the explanation. Nevertheless, these findings were very intriguing, and we decided to pursue this line of investigation. Gary Lynch, Christine Gall (Gary's long-time partner), Xiaoning and I submitted a large program project to the NIH, which included our 4 different laboratories to understand the links between the AMPA receptors, BDNF, synaptic plasticity and learning and memory. This project ended up being funded for the next 12 years. My laboratory focused on understanding how ampakine treatment could stimulate calpain and what could be the functional consequences of such activation for synaptic plasticity. As we will see later, this program turned out to be very successful and critical for our understanding of the roles of calpain-1 and calpain-2 in the brain.

As I kept reading the literature dealing with calpain, I came across a publication suggesting that calpain inhibitors could prevent the pathological changes in a mouse model of Parkinson's disease (PD)[7]. PD is a devastating neurodegenerative disease, which, like Alzheimer's disease, affects a large number of aged individuals. Like for AD, there is a small percentage of cases where the disease is caused by mutations in some genes, but the majority of cases is not due to any know mutations, and the disease is therefore called sporadic. This disease affects a particular type of neurons, the dopaminergic neurons, which are involved in the control of movement initiation. These neurons degenerate and this is one of the reasons PD patients exhibit tremor and have difficulties moving. Several animal models of the disease have been developed in mice and rats, each of these models with their own advantages and limitations. I mentioned earlier that Robert Siman, who had been a postdoc in Gary's lab when I was also still in the lab, had moved to Cephalon and developed a calpain inhibitor program there. He had generated a number of inhibitors and suggested I test these inhibitors in models of Parkinson's disease. I submitted a proposal to the NIH directed at testing the potential use of calpain inhibitors as treatment for Parkinson's disease. This proposal received funding from the NIH in 2006, although at the end of the 5-year project, we obtained mostly unconclusive results. Again, the reason for this lack of significant results became clearer several years later when we discovered that we needed to focus on selective calpain-2 inhibitors.

I had reached the end of my leave of absence, and I needed to go back to USC and restart my faculty position and my lab. Had Gary been successful in getting funding for Thorus, I might have been tempted to leave academia and to focus on doing translational research. However, as we discussed, Thorus was too early stage and Gary was not particularly interested in chasing investors to fund Thorus. Thus, in 2004, I left UCI and went back to work at USC.

Looking back at these 2 years spent at UCI, it looks like I did not accomplish much. However, when I analyze in more detail all the things I did, I can safely conclude that these were in fact very productive years.

- As VP Research at Tensor, I learned more about how to run research in a start-up company and to manage both financials and human resources. It also provided insight into the various ways to get the company funded and how to interact with potential sources of funding.
- Working with Cortex Pharmaceuticals was different since Cortex was already a publicly traded company, and the goals there were clearly to enhance the value of the existing assets of the company and to provide further evidence for the potential applications of the ampakine molecules for various therapeutic applications.

- On the scientific level, we made some very interesting discoveries with the finding that ampakine treatment of cultured hippocampal slices resulted in calpain activation without evidence of neurodegeneration. The link with BDNF, which we proposed to further analyze in the framework of a Program Project funded by the NIH would provide a critical piece of the puzzle to understand the roles of calpains in the brain. Thus, we had provided new scientific findings and obtained funding to continue this line of inquiry.
- Finally, on the personal level, I got married to a wonderful woman who became my inspiration, my collaborator and my strongest supporter. My children from my previous marriage became used to sharing the Friday afternoon pizza celebration at 101 Theory where all the various members of Tensor, Thorus and the academic personnel would come together and exchange their various results. It was time to turn the page and to start the next chapter of my quest to understand the functions of calpains in the brain.

Chapter 8
BACK TO USC

After my 2 years period with Gary at UCI, it was time for me to return to USC at the end of 2003. I was fortunate to be able to rebuild a strong research team thanks to the funding from the NIH and also DARPA, as Ted Berger and I succeeded in getting a large grant to use hippocampal slices as a potential tool to detect environmental threats (this was obviously following the 2001 attack on the US). The idea was relatively similar to what Tensor Pharmaceuticals was doing and consisted in using the patterns of electrical activity recorded in hippocampal slices placed on multielectrode arrays as an assay for detecting and classifying specific classes of molecules. This work got the attention of the local media, and I was interviewed by Channel 9. The reporter and a crew from Channel 9 spent almost 3 hours filming and talking to me about our work. The evening the interview was scheduled to be aired on Channel 9, I waited anxiously in front of my television, as I thought it would be shown on the 7:00pm show. It was not. When it finally came on after 9:00pm, Xiaoning had already fallen asleep, and she missed my moment of fame.... This made me realize that an interview which lasted about 3 hours ended up in a 20-second piece in the evening news.

The progress of molecular biology in the late 80s/early 90s led to the development of very powerful tools to better understand the functions of specific genes and proteins. In particular, the ability to selectively turn off or to insert genes in mice has generated a huge number of mutant mice that lack or overexpress proteins of interest[1]. It was with great excitement that we found out in early 2000 that a laboratory at Tufts University in Boston had generated a mutant mouse lacking one of the isoforms of calpains, calpain-1. Dr. Chishti was interested in understanding the role of calpain-1 in blood platelets, these tiny blood cells that form clots to stop bleeding. In 2001, his lab published the first manuscript using a calpain-1 knock-out mouse to reveal an essential role for calpain-1 in platelet function[2]. I immediately contacted Dr. Chishti and asked him if I could use his mutant mice to study the role of calpain-1 in synaptic plasticity and learning and memory. Dr. Chishti agreed to provide my lab with a small number of mutant mice and their respective control mice, also called wild-type mice. I was beyond excited by the prospect that these mice would provide the definitive proof of the validity of the 1984 hypothesis, as I was certain that these mice would show impairment in both synaptic plasticity and learning and memory. I convinced a graduate student in the lab, Michael Grammer, to take on this project and told him that the results of these experiments would make him famous. As it happened, it did not turn out so well. He first tested these mice, which we finally received after multiple discussions with Dr. Chishti in 2004, for their ability to learn an association between a sound and a foot-shock. For this test, mice are placed in a cage with a grid floor and are exposed to a tone followed by a mild electric shock to their paws, which makes the mice jump to avoid the shock. The following day, mice are placed in the same cage and the memory of the painful experience from the previous day makes the mice "freeze", meaning they stop moving (Fig. 1). The duration of the freezing during a 5-min observation time is a good index of the strength of the memory, as mice with little memory do not freeze, while mice with long freezing times are assumed to have a strong memory of the painful experience. When Michael tested the calpain-1 knock-out mice, they showed the same degree of freezing as the corresponding mice with normal calpain-1. He then used hippocampal slices from the same mice to determine the magnitude of the

LTP phenomenon in response to a specific pattern of electrical stimulation, which Gary's lab had shown to be the optimal pattern to elicit LTP and which he called the theta burst stimulation (TBS), meaning that short pulses of electrical stimulation delivered at 100 Hz were repeated a few times at the theta frequency (5-7 Hz).

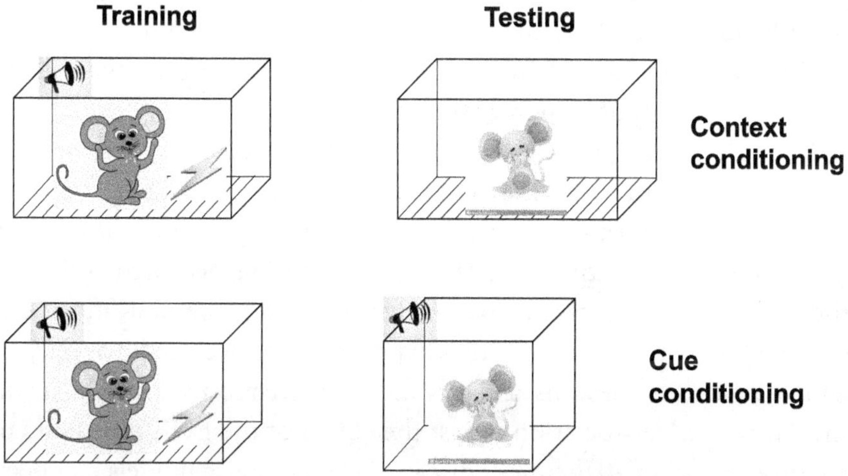

Figure 1: Schematic representation of fear conditioning. On day 1, mice are exposed to a tone and to a foot-shock (training). On day 2, they are placed in the same box and the duration of freezing is recorded. The memory of the context where the shock was received evokes a fear response (freezing). On day 3, mice are placed in a different box and are exposed to the tone. The memory of the tone evokes a fear response.

As mentioned before, the theta frequency is the frequency observed in the electroencephalogram (EEG) of animals and humans exploring a new environment and is thought to be used to facilitate the storage of new information in the brain. To my great sorrow, the LTP magnitude in the calpain-1 knock-out mice was identical to that found in the mice with normal calpain-1.

I was devastated, and for many days I could not believe the results, which contradicted more than 20 years of my previous research. This was one of those moments that make you seriously doubt yourself and your faith in the scientific process. I almost wanted to quit doing research at this point. After about a week, I started to recover and to go back to the drawing board and to think about an alternative explanation. Furthermore, to enable Michael Grammer to complete his dissertation, I agreed to publish the negative results he had obtained with these mice, something that would haunt me for many years[3]. By doing so, I was publicly acknowledging that we had been wrong all these years and that calpain-1 had nothing to do with synaptic plasticity and learning. On the other hand, this result implied that calpain was perhaps more important for neurodegeneration than for plasticity and learning. As we will see later, this was only a temporary setback.

I was also pursuing the work with Eukarion molecules, and we were quite successful in demonstrating that these molecules had potentially great value. The idea that oxygen free radicals play a significant role in many neurodegenerative disorders was already well accepted, although the evidence for that was not extremely convincing. The EUK molecules provided a great tool to test this hypothesis and we used a variety of animal models of these diseases to validate it. We received funding from the Alzheimer's Association to test the effects of the EUK molecules in a mouse model of Alzheimer's disease. Several mouse models had been developed at various institutions. In particular, one mouse model had been developed at UC Irvine, and we were able to obtain the mice from Dr. Frank LaFerla, the scientist who had developed this model[4]. As we mentioned before, a small fraction of AD patients have some mutations in a few genes, and the disease is then called familial AD, as opposed to the majority of patients with no known mutations and the disease is then called sporadic. The model that Frank LaFerla had developed exhibited three of the mutations found in familial AD, and the mice were therefore called the 3xAD mice or 3xTgAD[4]. These mice developed normally and were able to reproduce just like normal mice. However, as they become older, they started to exhibit many of the pathological manifestations found in the human disease, except for the neurodegeneration. They have amyloid plaques, which are aggregates of the famous ß-amyloid peptide, as well as neurofibrillary tangles, which are aggregates of hyperphosphorylated tau protein. Finally, they also exhibit cognitive impairment. We showed that in the 3xTgAD mouse model of Alzheimer's disease, a chronic treatment with EUK-207 for 5 months starting in mice aged 4-month-old, which did not exhibit any significant signs of pathology, could prevent the appearance of most of the pathological features of the disease, including the plaques and tangles (Fig. 2), as well as the cognitive decline[5].

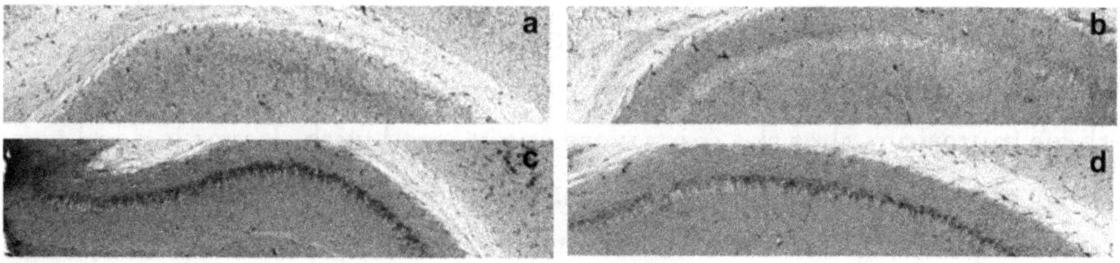

Figure 2: Effects of EUK-207 on neurofibrillary tangles in the 3xTg mice.

Wild-type and 3xTG mice were treated with vehicle or with EUK-207 for 5 months starting at 4 months of age. Brains were sectioned and sections were stained for a marker of neurofibrillary tangles. a: wild type treated with vehicle. b: wild-type treated with EUK-207. c: 3xTgAD treated with vehicle. d: 3xTgAD treated with EUK-207. Note the large increase in staining for neurofibrillary tangles in the 3xTgAD section (compare c to a) and the reduction in the staining for neurofibrillary tangles with EUK-207 treatment (compare d to c). From Clausen et al.[5].

Furthermore, a 3-month treatment with EUK-207 starting in mice aged 9-month-old, which therefore exhibited significant signs of the disease, was also able to prevent the development of the pathology and the cognitive decline. These results provided strong evidence that oxygen free radicals do play a very significant role in the development of AD pathology. Encouraged by these results, we decided to test the effects of the EUK molecules in normal aging, since there was already a significant body of evidence that accumulation of free radicals also participated in the aging process. Interestingly, a 6-month treatment of mice aged 16-month-old with either Euk-189 or Euk-207 was able to reverse oxidative stress and cognitive decline[6]. Thus, not only did our results provide clear evidence for a critical role of oxygen free radicals in age-related diseases, but they also suggested that SOD-catalase mimetics could become useful therapeutic treatments for such diseases. As discussed earlier, we were unfortunately not able to bring them to the clinic. One difficulty for the clinical development of these molecules was due to the fact that these molecules were not orally active, as they fall apart in the stomach due to the acidic pH. Another reason was that the mouse model we used is poorly predictive of the effects of drugs in humans. As has been said repeatedly, scientists have cured AD 100 times in mice but none of the tested treatments have shown significant effects in human patients. The model we used has also been criticized on the basis that there is no human patient who is exhibiting all the three mutations that the mice were engineered with. It was indeed very unfortunate that we could not bring these molecules to the clinic, as there are now many ways to resolve the delivery problems for promising molecules. In particular, novel intranasal delivery technologies are being increasingly used to avoid the issue of oral availability, especially for drugs targeting the brain. We can only hope that it might be possible at some future time to test the possibility of using intranasal delivery of these EUK molecules for the treatment of age-related neurodegenerative diseases.

You may remember that I had started Rhenovia in 2007 and I would go to Mulhouse at least 3 times a year to review the progress we were making in developing computational tools to understand the interactions between drugs and neural networks. This involved the collaboration between a team at USC, which included Ted Berger and one of my former Ph.D. students, Jean-Marie Bouteiller, who was working as a postdoc with Ted, and the Rhenovia team in Mulhouse. The beauty of computational models is that they do not require animal experimentation; most experiments are very quick (once the program has been generated) and provide amazing results which do not need multiple replications.

Figure 3 shows some results obtained using a relatively simple model of the NMDA receptors with open and close states to illustrate the power of the simulation and the ability to reproduce very closely some experimental data. We developed a very sophisticated model of a glutamatergic synapse, similar to what was shown in Figure 4, Chapter 2. Using this model, we were able to provide a very detailed and quantitative analysis of the interactions between the AMPA and the NMDA receptors (Fig. 4).

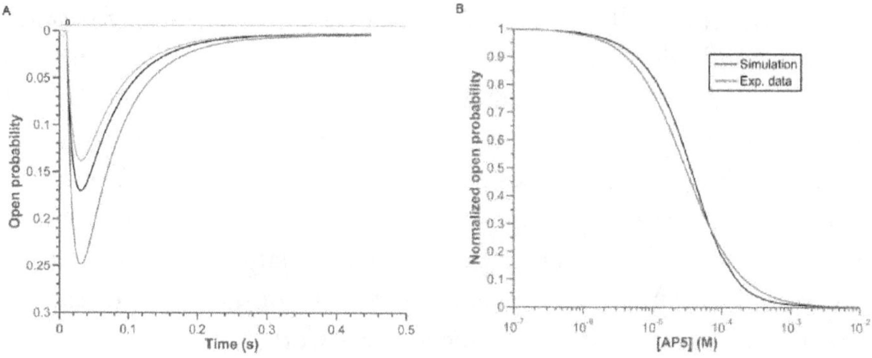

Figure 3: Computer simulations of the NMDA receptor.

a. Open probability of the NMDA receptor in response to a brief application of 1 mM glutamate for 4 msec in the absence or presence of 20 μM of the NMDA receptor antagonist, AP5 (black line) or 30 μM AP5 (green line).
b. Maximum open probability of the NMDA receptor in the presence of different concentrations of AP5. Experimental data from Harrison et al (1985) (red line); simulated data (black line). Adapted from Ambert et al,[7].

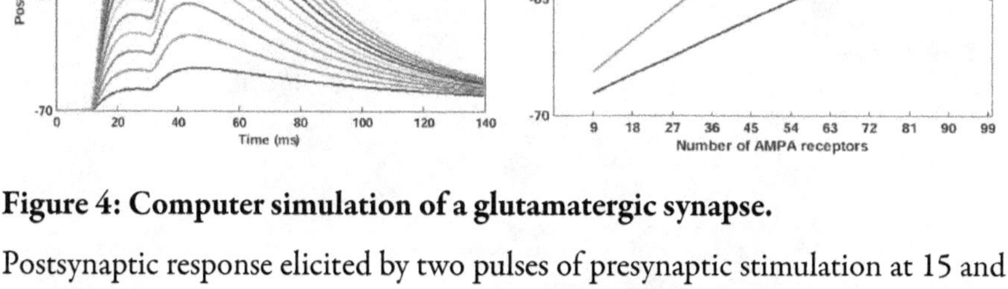

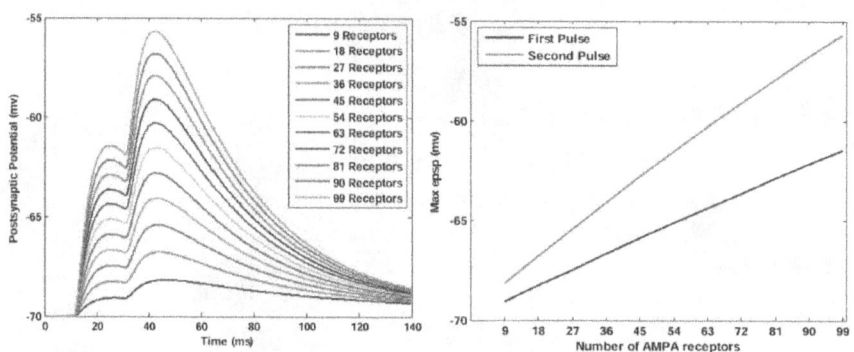

Figure 4: Computer simulation of a glutamatergic synapse.

Postsynaptic response elicited by two pulses of presynaptic stimulation at 15 and 30 msec. The model simulates the responses at synapses with increasing number of AMPA receptors from 9 to 99 receptors (left). The postsynaptic response increases linearly with the number of AMPA receptors but the increase is larger for the second pulse as compared to the first pulse, due to the activation of a larger fraction of the receptors. (Adapted from Bouteiller et al,[8]).

These brief results illustrate the power of this approach. The computer can run hundreds of experiments each day, which would take months to run in the lab. One can therefore screen the effects of large numbers of molecules on synaptic responses, as long as some parameters are available to include in the program. We even reached the point that the program could simulate not only events at the molecular level, but also events at the network level, simulating the activities of large numbers of excitatory and inhibitory neurons and reproducing a multitude of experimental results. We also spent almost a year working for free for Pfizer, which had a group devoted to computational neuroscience, but they were not able to decide how to collaborate with us. As we mentioned above, we were not able to attract the interest of pharma companies or other potential investors to pursue this approach at Rhenovia, and Rhenovia had to close doors in 2015. As discussed previously, such approach is now much more applied by both academic labs and pharmaceutical companies, as it eliminates the sometime controversial use of animals, and considerably speeds up the drug discovery process.

Chapter 9
RENEWING WITH SUCCESS

In 2004 a very talented graduate student, Wei Xu, started his Ph.D. studies in my lab at USC. Wei was a unique student, as he had already completed a master's degree in Canada before starting his Ph.D. program. He rapidly designed his research project, which involved investigating whether a third type of glutamate receptors, the so-called glutamate metabotropic receptor, could also be cleaved by calpain the same way we had showed for the other 2 types of glutamate receptors, the AMPA and NMDA receptors, were cleaved. Not only did Wei find that it was indeed the case, but he decided to further investigate whether the truncated receptor had a different function than the intact receptor. And indeed, what he found was quite remarkable. While the intact receptor has a neuroprotective function in neurons, the truncated receptor switched its function to become neurodegenerative (Fig. 1).

Wei went on to demonstrate that this mechanism was taking place in the intact animal following seizure activity, which represents uncontrolled exuberant activity of neuronal networks, similar to what takes place in humans with epilepsy. Following seizure activity, the metabotropic glutamate receptor was indeed cleaved by calpain. Wei devised a clever way to prevent this truncation by using an engineered small

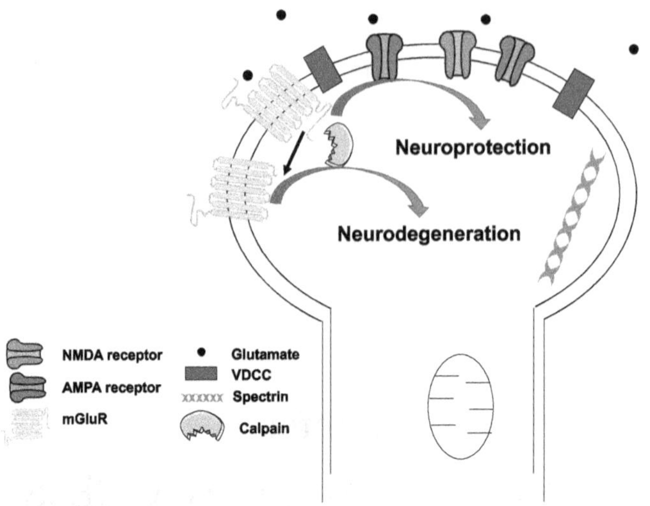

Figure 1: Calpain-mediated truncation of the mGluR switches its function from neuroprotective to neurodegenerative. Calpain activation following an influx of calcium in the dendritic spine results in the truncation of the N-terminal domain of the mGluR. This switches the function of the receptor from neuroprotection to neurodegeneration[1].

peptide and showed that this peptide when injected in the animal following seizures was able to prevent the truncation of the receptor and the neuronal damage resulting from this truncation. It was also able to provide neuroprotection in a rat model of ischemia in the postnatal period[2]. All these results were strong evidence supporting a role of calpain in neurodegeneration, a topic we had started back in the 80s, and had led to the creation of Cortex Pharmaceuticals.

As has been said before, the scientific enterprise is really a teamwork, and requires the participation of many students, postdocs and faculty. It also requires a continuous reading of the literature, as findings in other fields not necessarily related to the field of interest could have direct relevance to a particular question. This is why the American universities are so powerful in science, as they house the best libraries in the world. When I first came from France to UC Irvine, I would spend at least 2 hours every morning in the library reading the latest scientific journals. We did not have the computers then that we have today, and I would make photocopies of every article I found interesting. I filled up boxes and boxes of such copies, which I religiously moved from UCI to USC when I left UCI. I continued the process after I arrived at USC, since by then, we still did not have internet, and the desktop computers had very little storage capacity. By the time I left USC, I had an entire room filled with photocopies. By then, I decided to get rid of them all, since we had internet and unlimited access to all the journals, and the computers could store thousands of manuscripts. Nowadays, this sort of activity is archaic since all researchers can directly access all the publications directly from their own computers. I keep telling my students how lucky they are to have this unlimited access to the literature and that they must take advantage of this tool to design their experiments and to write their manuscripts. On the other hand, as has been also discussed extensively, there are now so many journals and so many publications that it is impossible to read all the papers on a particular topic.

Such reading made me realize that, in certain tissues, calpain-2, the calpain variant that we thought could not be activated by calcium under normal conditions, could be activated almost in the absence of calcium by a phosphorylation event, the addition of a phosphate group to specific side chains in the protein. This had been shown in epithelial cells (the cells that make the skin) following treatment with a growth factor, the epithelial growth factor (EGF), which stimulated the activity of a protein kinase, an enzyme that catalyzes the addition of a phosphate group to a protein[3]. In all proteins, addition of such a group results in a change in the 3-D conformation of the protein and therefore in a change in its function.

We immediately wanted to test whether brain calpain-2 could also get activated by such a phosphorylation event following treatment of brain slices with either EGF or BDNF (the growth factor mentioned previously). Another talented graduate student, Sohila Zadran, took the project in her hands and ran with it. In less than 2 years, she showed indeed that calpain-2 could very well be the variant of calpain involved in synaptic plasticity. She found that BDNF activated calpain-2 in dendrites in and dendritic spines, even in the absence of calcium[4], and this effect was also associated with the polymerization of actin into actin filaments, an event widely recognized to participate in the structural reorganization implicated in synaptic plasticity (Fig. 2)[5].

This result was hugely important, as it removed a major obstacle in our way of thinking of the role of calpain-2 in synaptic plasticity. As discussed earlier, calpain-1 is normally activated by very low concentrations of calcium whereas calpain-2 requires much higher calcium concentrations, which are probably never observed under normal physiological conditions. This had led us and most researchers in the field to the idea that it should be calpain-1, which was involved in synaptic plasticity and not calpain-2. These new findings from the literature and our own experiments indicated that this assumption could be wrong, as calpain-2 could be activated through a mechanism that did not require a large influx of calcium.

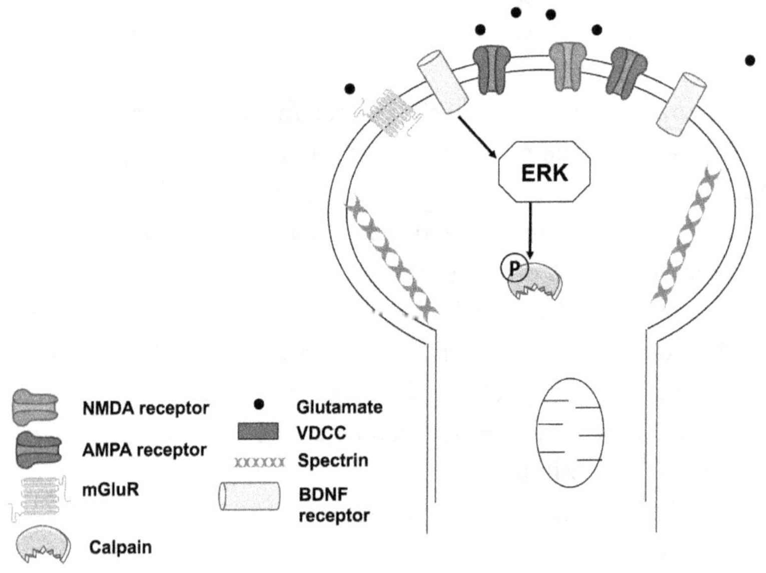

Figure 2: Link between BDNF and calpain.

BDNF stimulation of its receptor leads to activation of a protein kinase, called ERK, which phosphorylates calpain-2 and activates it.

As BDNF had been shown to be involved in synaptic plasticity, we were very quick to postulate that this suggested that calpain-2 was also involved in synaptic plasticity. This result also provided an explanation for the phenomenon we had discovered when I went back to UCI, which was that ampakines could activate calpain in hippocampal slices. As we discussed earlier, we had also found that ampakines could increase the levels of BDNF. Thus, there was now a clear link between ampakines, BDNF and calpain activation. This led to several publications, as well as to the scientific writer at USC to write a story with the title "Memory molecule, Déjà vu", as our findings were published 26 years after our original Science paper. We were back full steam working on the original hypothesis concerning the critical role of calpain in synaptic plasticity and learning and memory. However, we still did not get it, as we thought that calpain-2 was the calpain variant that could be involved in our original 1984 hypothesis. But this turned out to be wrong too.

At the end of 2010, my wife, Xiaoning Bi, who had taken a position at Western University of Health Sciences (WesternU) in Pomona, CA, told me that WesternU was initiating a search for the Dean of the Graduate College of Biomedical Sciences. We discussed this opportunity, and we decided that I should apply for the position. I had previously given a seminar at WesternU and, since Xiaoning was working there, I had a pretty good idea of what was going on there. Pomona is not very far from downtown Los Angeles, and it was quite easy to spend time talking to the members of the search committee and to the Provost and the President of WesternU. I clearly had an edge since I had met many of the people involved at some of the social events Xiaoning had brought me with her. Following the usual process of interviewing, I was offered the position. I talked to Richard Thompson, my mentor at USC and asked his advice. What he said made a strong impression on me; basically, he used the model of UCI and pointed out that an initial small number of talented faculty in the Department of Psychobiology was able to have a huge impact in the field of learning and memory. In other words, he told me that if I could recruit a few talented faculty members at WesternU, I could also have a huge impact on neurosciences. This was a very strong incentive. In addition, WesternU offered me significant incentives to make the move more attractive. I was also drawn by the prospect of having a significant impact on the research and training of students at WesternU, since the provost was particularly interested in having me starting a Ph.D. program at WesternU. Another strong motivating factor was that my wife Xiaoning was already working there and was now a Full Professor in the College of Osteopathic Medicine. The idea of having a lab next to my wife's lab, and to be able to collaborate on a daily basis was very attractive. Before that, we would often carry biological samples between her or my lab and store them in our home fridge before taking them back to our respective labs. On the other hand, I had a wonderful collaboration with Ted Berger, and we were awarded a large grant from the NIH to use computational and experimental approaches to better understand the mechanisms of learning and memory. We were also working together for Rhenovia, the company I had started with Serge Bischoff in Mulhouse, and I was still naively convinced that we could make Rhenovia the Google of the computational neuroscience companies. Despite all this, I ultimately decided to take the position of Dean of the Graduate College of Biomedical Sciences and to move my lab to Pomona.

It is interesting to compare the logos and mottos of the various institutions I have been trained or worked in (Fig. 3). As previously mentioned, the one from the Ecole Polytechnique left a profound impression on me, and I think I have been faithful to this motto by strongly following the pursuit of sciences, hoping it would lead me to glory. The motto of the University of California is much simpler but also represents a strong stimulus for the pursuit of truth and knowledge, and again, I believe I did follow the right path. The motto from USC is much more esoteric and is open to several interpretations. One of these reflects the tradition of giving the victorious gladiator a palm branch as a reward. I guess I am still in pursuit of victory and the coming years might determine if I succeed or not. Finally, I am convinced that I am following WesternU's motto to the letter, as I went there to teach, to do research to increase our scientific knowledge, and to develop a treatment to protect and heal the damaged brain.

By the end of 2011, I had spent 23 years at USC and had made lots of friends and colleagues, and it was difficult to leave them behind. I had trained 10 postdocs, 28 graduate students and published 230 manuscripts. Following the example of my friend Bernard Malfroy I had even run the LA Marathon about 10 times, as it was quite convenient since the departure and arrival of the race was at the Coliseum then. I could come to my office in the Hedco building early before the departure time of the marathon to change into my running clothes, and to get ready for the run. After the race, I would just return to my office and recover before driving back home.

Ecole Polytechnique

POUR LA PATRIE LES SCIENCES ET LA GLOIRE
For Fatherland, sciences and glory

UC Irvine

LET THERE BE LIGHT

University of Southern California

PALMAM QUI MERUIT FERAT
Let whoever earns the palm bear it

Western University of Health Sciences

Western University OF HEALTH SCIENCES

Educare, Sanare, Coniunctim
To teach to heal together

Figure 3: Logos and mottos from the various institutions I was trained in and worked for.

More importantly, I had continued to make significant contributions to the field of calpains and demonstrated that calpain played significant roles in the regulation of synaptic transmission and in neurodegeneration. I had solved the paradox regarding the physiological activation of calpain-2, despite its high calcium requirement, and was getting closer to understanding its functions. On the other hand, I had found that calpain-1 might not be involved in synaptic plasticity and learning and memory, which was still a very sore aspect of my work at USC. I had started two biotech companies, Eukarion and Rhenovia, although Eukarion had not succeeded in bringing its molecules to the clinic. Rhenovia was still running, and we were making great progress in developing an amazing tool to understand the ways drugs could interact with neural networks. My lab had been continuously funded by the NIH and other sources of funding. But I still did not solve the puzzle regarding what calpain-1 and calpain-2 were doing in the brain. This was going to happen in the next stage of my career.

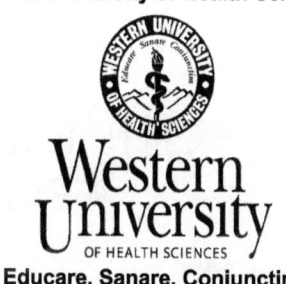

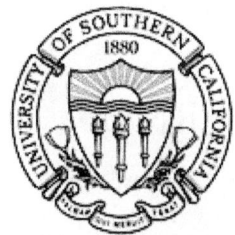

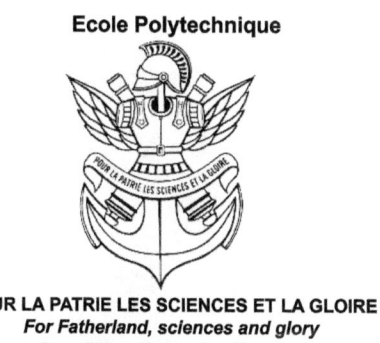

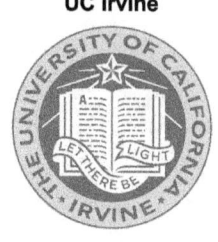

Chapter 10
THE EARLY WESTERNU YEARS: 2012-2016

It is often said that moving is both stressful and exhilarating. Stressful because one is starting in a new environment with new people, new rules and new expectations. Exhilarating because it opens new opportunities and acts like a rebirth. I was truly excited to move my lab from USC to WesternU (Fig. 1).

I was fortunate that I could take with me a few people from my USC lab who agreed to help with the move and to set up the new lab. USC was also quite generous as I was able to take with me a lot of equipment and supplies, which I had accumulated over my 23 years of work there. In fact, we needed 3 large trucks full of materials to move everything from USC to Pomona. Quite remarkably, it took us less than a week to set up the lab and to start running experiments in the new lab. Moreover, the stars were aligned for me as I was able to recruit three very talented post-docs. One of the first things I did when I went to Pomona was to ask Dr. Chishti if I could get the calpain-1 knock-out mice again, but this time I established my own mouse colony to make sure I had complete control of the mice and of their genotype. I really wanted to go back to try to repeat the experiments we had done at USC, which resulted in negative

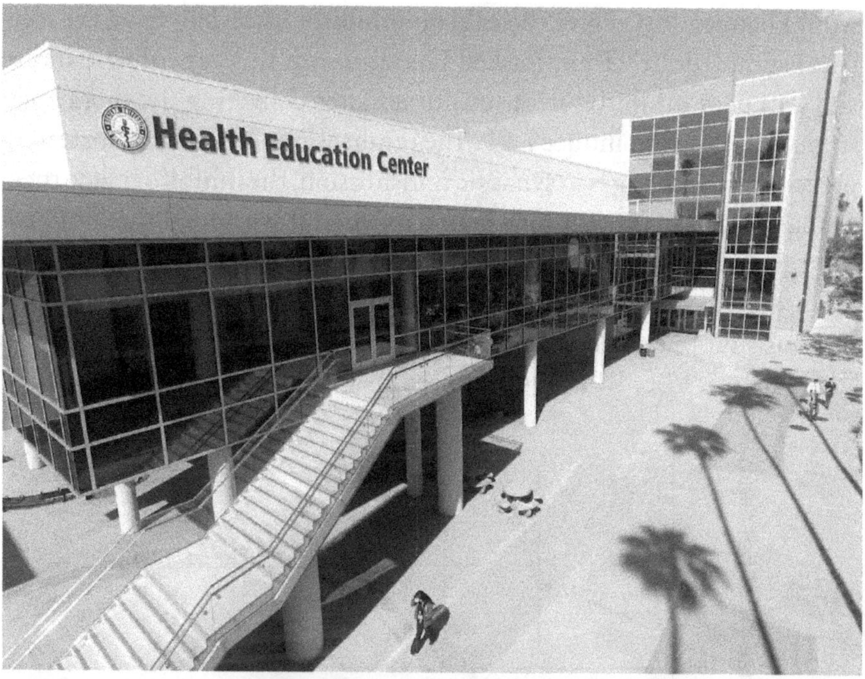

Figure 1: The Health Education Center (HEC) building at Western University of Health Sciences. Western University of Health Sciences is located downtown Pomona in what used to be a shopping mall in the 70s. It has expanded considerably since its creation in 1977 and has an enrollment of over 3,500 students. My laboratory is located on the 4th floor of the building, which is devoted to research.

results. I guess I still did not believe that the results we had obtained were a true reflection of the function of calpain-1. I also asked one of my new postdocs, Dr. Guoqi Zu, to perform an experiment that had been suggested by a researcher at UCLA, Dr. David Glanzman, when I gave a seminar there.

As the reader may remember, our original hypothesis regarding the role of calpain in synaptic plasticity was in part due to the finding that inhibiting calpain could prevent activity-dependent changes in synaptic plasticity in experiments performed with hippocampal slices[1]. In these experiments, we added the calpain inhibitor to the medium bathing the slices before delivering the electrical stimuli producing the changes in synaptic transmission. What the UCLA scientist asked me was "what would happen if you give the calpain inhibitor after delivering the electrical stimulation?" Thus, I asked Guoqi to run this experiment and to add a calpain inhibitor at various times after delivering the theta burst stimulation used to induce LTP. The results were astonishing! Instead of preventing the changes in synaptic transmission, the inhibitor made these changes even larger! But that only happened if we added the inhibitor in a time window between 5 and 45 min after the electrical stimulation. If we waited one hour, nothing happened and the changes in synaptic transmission remained stable (Fig. 2). When the calpain inhibitor was added before TBS, LTP was inhibited, as we had observed previously[2].

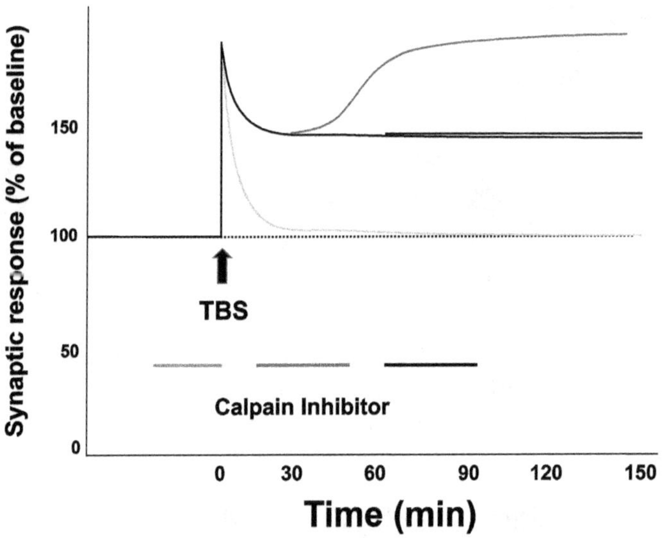

Figure 2: Different effects of a non-selective calpain inhibitor on LTP at different time points.

Hippocampal slices were incubated in the presence of a calpain inhibitor added at different times before or after delivering the theta burst stimulation to elicit LTP: for 20 min before TBS, for 30 min 10 min after TBS or for 30 min 1 h after TBS (modified from Wang et al.[2]).

This was one of these Eureka moments, which happen rarely but completely change the way one thinks about a particular question. When I told these results to Gary, he was also amazed but he quickly realized that it was in good agreement with some of the most recent results his lab had obtained, which suggested that synapses in the hippocampus exist in various states, with some synapses more easily potentiated than others. What he suggested to account for our results was that inhibiting calpain after TBS could lower the threshold for potentiation of synapses with a high threshold for potentiation. This did not turn out to be correct.

During the same period, we received the calpain-1 knock-out mice from Dr. Chishti and started a breeding colony. The same postdoc, Guoqi, performed the LTP experiment we had done at USC with the new mice, and we got another surprising result. This time, we did find the expected results, as these mice showed no LTP following the delivery of the theta-burst stimulation. Moreover, these mice also showed an impairment in learning and memory, when we trained them in the fear conditioning paradigm[3]. Guoqi was very careful and paid close attention to all the details of the experiments. He figured out why the previous experiments, which had a few variations in some of the parameters, did not work. When he used the same parameters that Michael Grammer had used, he did replicate his result. Because the mice we got at USC were older than the ones we generally used, Michael had changed some of the parameters for the electrical stimulation (he increased the intensity of the stimulation he was using during TBS), and these changes were sufficient to change the results. Likewise, when we tested the learning in the fear conditioning paradigm at USC, the calpain-1 knock-out mice did not exhibit a learning impairment. Again, the parameters that Michael Grammer used were slightly different than the ones we normally used. These results therefore completely confirmed that calpain-1 activation was necessary for triggering LTP and for episodic learning.

Interestingly, Guoqi tried a different stimulation protocol to elicit LTP, which has also been used frequently in different labs. Instead of using the theta burst stimulation, he used a 1 sec of stimulation at 100 Hz. This protocol was routinely used before Gary discovered that the optimal stimulation protocol was the theta burst stimulation. Surprisingly, LTP elicited by this protocol was perfectly normal in the calpain-1 knock-out mice. These results revealed that different types of electrical stimulation can induced the same LTP but by activating different signaling pathways[4]. Likewise, different training protocols could produce similar learning by engaging different signaling pathways. We think that this is probably the explanation for the differential effects of a calpain inhibitor on various forms of learning we discussed previously. And these results also suggested that there are multiple ways to modify the strength of synaptic contacts and to store new information. This should not be a surprise, since these processes are the results of thousands of years of evolution and, as had been discussed many times, biology does not mind redundancy if it leads to the right endpoints. But then, it remained to explain the increase in LTP magnitude when the added the calpain inhibitor after the electrical stimulation.

You may remember that we had found that the growth factor BDNF was able to stimulate calpain-2 in hippocampus. BDNF had also been shown to be released from neurons following the electrical stimulation that elicits LTP. We then thought that the activation of calpain-2 following BDNF release could be responsible for limiting the extent of LTP, and if this was true, then calpain-2 inhibition after theta-burst stimulation would indeed result in an enhancement of LTP.

To really confirm this new hypothesis, we needed an inhibitor that could selectively inhibit calpain-2. This is where the story goes back to the creation of Cortex Pharmaceuticals by Gary Lynch in the 80s. Cortex Pharmaceuticals had recruited a chemist from Georgia Tech to synthesize a large number of calpain inhibitors. We went back to the publications and patents produced by this chemist and identified one molecule that had a much better selectivity for calpain-2 than for calpain-1. We contacted this chemist, and he sent us 5 mg of this molecule, we refer to as C2I (calpain-2 inhibitor) and sometimes as NA-101. Sure enough, this molecule worked as predicted. It did not affect the triggering of the changes in synaptic plasticity when applied before the train of electrical stimulation but enhanced the amplitude of the changes in synaptic transmission elicited by TBS. It also enhanced the magnitude of LTP when added after the theta-burst stimulation and did not do anything if applied 1 h after TBS[2]. Moreover, this selective calpain-2 inhibitor also facilitated learning in the fear conditioning paradigm in normal mice[5]. We finally got it right! This was 30 years after Gary and I had published our hypothesis in *Science*. I submitted the manuscript to Science thinking that the journal would be interested in these findings, which provided definitive proof for our hypothesis, but for some unknown reason, Science was not interested. Our hypothesis regarding the roles of calpain-1 and calpain-2 in LTP is schematized in Figure 3. In our model, TBS would activate calpain-1 in selected dendritic spines, leading to LTP. On the other hand, calpain-2 activation in neighboring dendritic spines would prevent LTP developing in these spines.

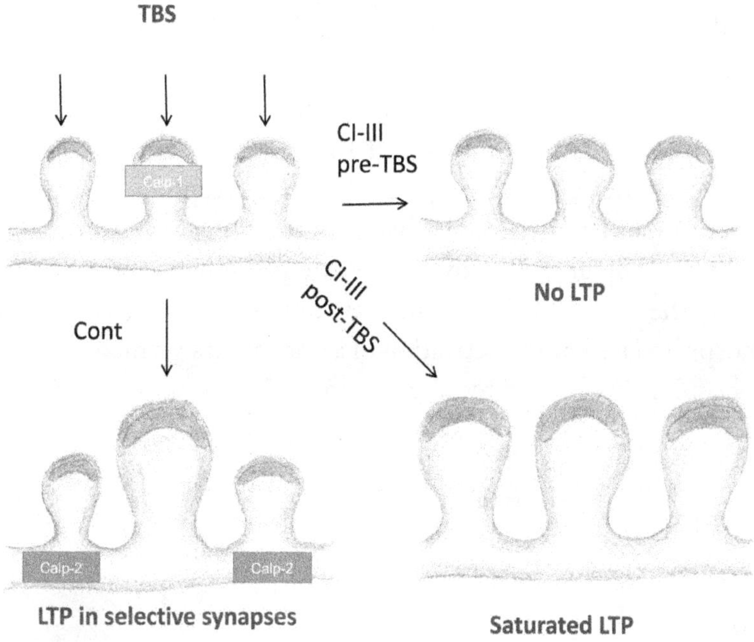

Figure 3: Roles of calpain-1 and calpain-2 in LTP.

TBS activates calpain-1 in selected dendritic spines, thus leading to LTP formation. Addition of a calpain-1 inhibitor before TBS would block LTP formation. On the other hand, calpain-2 activation in neighboring dendritic spines would prevent LTP formation. Addition of a calpain inhibitor after TBS or of a selective calpain-2 inhibitor before TBS would result in LTP formation in all the dendritic spines activated (modified from Wang et al.[2]).

Again, it is worth stressing that these results were indeed quite remarkable. While calpain-1 activation was required to initiate certain types of synaptic plasticity and certain forms of learning, calpain-2 activation in the minutes following the presentation of the information limited the extent of changes in synaptic strength and the extent of learning.

When we published our findings, we entitled our manuscript "A molecular brake controls the magnitude of long-term potentiation." We also used a number of approaches to analyze the time-course of activation of calpain-1 and calpain-2 following the delivery of the electrical stimulation. Our results are summarized in Fig. 4 and indicated that calpain-1 was rapidly but transiently activated following TBS, with a peak of activation probably within 1 minute and a return to silent mode (recall that calpain-1 activation requires calcium) by 2-3 minutes. In contrast, calpain-2 activation would start after 1 minute but lasts for about 45 minutes with a return to inactivated status by 60 minutes. These time-courses are consistent with the fact that calpain-1 is activated by the rapid influx of calcium through the NMDA receptor/channel, which produces a rapid and transient change in the concentration of calcium. In contrast, calpain-2 is activated by the phosphorylation event triggered by the action of BDNF and remains activated until calpain-2 is dephosphorylated by the activation of a phosphatase, which will remove the phosphate group and terminate calpain-2 activation.

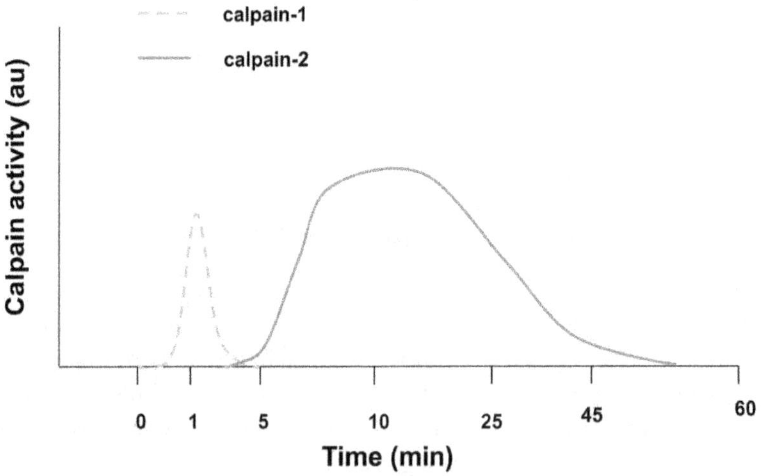

Figure 4: Schematic representation of the time-course for calpain-1 and calpain-2 activation following TBS.

Calpain-1 is rapidly but transiently activated by the influx of calcium provided by the stimulation of the synaptic NMDA receptors. Calpain-2 activation is delayed and lasts up to 45 minutes and is triggered by ERK-mediated phosphorylation due to the activation of the BDNF receptor.

Again, it is worth stressing the implications of these results and the fact that it took me almost 40 years to understand the roles of calpains in learning and memory. We started with the simple notion that calpain activation was necessary for triggering synaptic plasticity and consequently certain forms of learning. The story was in fact much more complicated and interesting, since we discovered that it was calpain-1 activation that was responsible for stimulating the cascade of events leading to synaptic reorganization and storing new information. The completely novel mechanism we had discovered was that calpain-2 activation shortly after calpain-1 activation limits how many synapses can be modified during the exposure to a new information, thereby limiting the extent of information that can be acquired at a given time. The question of why we cannot store every new piece of information has long been debated by psychologists, neurobiologists and clinicians. In his book "The mind of a mnemonist"[6], Alexander Luria describes the experience of S., who has an extraordinary memory but cannot make discriminations. Likewise, the movie "Rain Man" was based on the story of Kim Peek, who had a phenomenal memory but was living with the savant syndrome and could not survive without his father[7]. On the other hand, there are clearly many examples of people with exceptional memory who are living perfectly normal lives. It is perhaps another case of too much or not enough of a good thing.

What our studies revealed was that a selective calpain-2 inhibitor at the right dose might be able to enhance learning and provide significant benefit. Indeed, we showed that a selective calpain-2 inhibitor could facilitate learning in normal mice as well as in mice exhibiting impaired learning, such as the calpain-1 knock-out mice (Fig. 5)[5].

In recent experiments with a collaborator at Yale University, Dr. Amy Arnsten, we found that a single injection of a selective calpain-2 inhibitor to aged monkeys results in enhanced learning performance, indicating that this mechanism is present in non-human primates. As we are preparing human studies with a selective calpain-2 inhibitor, we will determine whether such an inhibitor can enhance learning in normal subjects as well as in subjects with impaired learning.

It is an interesting question to ask why the system has evolved such a complicated machinery to modify synaptic strength throughout

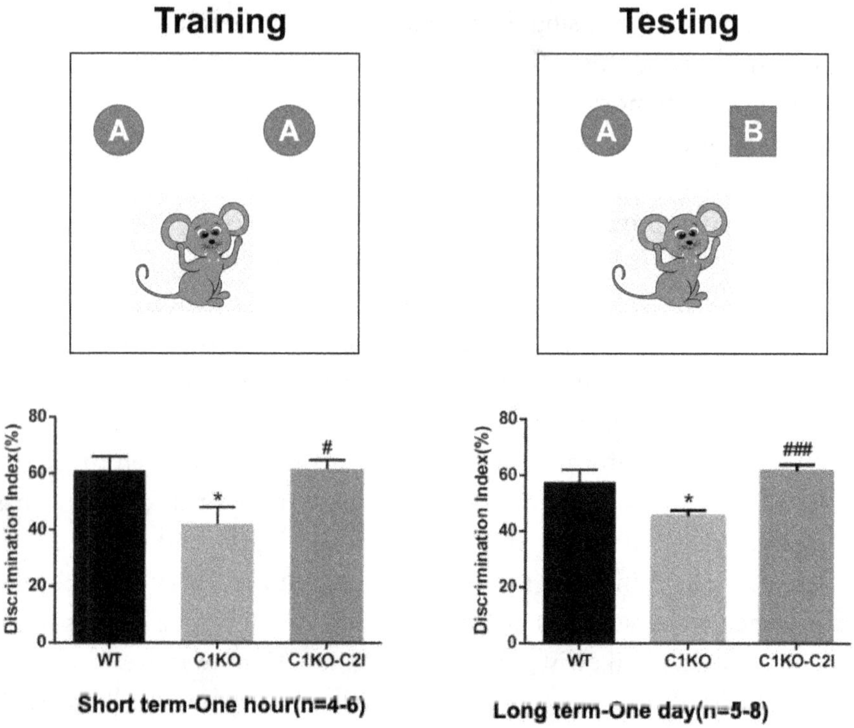

Figure 5: C2I (NA-101) reverses the learning impairment in calpain-1 knock-out mice.

Mice are placed in an arena and are exposed to two identical objects (A-A) they can explore freely. One hour or 24 hours later, they are reintroduced to the arena and are exposed to the same plus a new object (A-B). Normal mice will spend more time exploring the new object both at 1 hour and 24 hours later. Calpain-1 knock-outs are impaired and spend similar amount of time exploring both objects. Treatment with C2I/NA-101 30 min before training restores both short-term and long-term memory in the calpain-1 knock-out mice (modified from Liu et al., 2016[5]).

evolution. Xiaoning and I tried to provide some answers to this question, and we postulated that a potential explanation could be found in the mechanisms regulating cell motility[8]. We argued that many of the same processes that control cell motility have been used by cells, and in particular by neurons, to regulate a variety of cellular functions. In the model we proposed, calpain-1 was involved in promoting the formation of pseudopodia, which would stimulate the migration of cells in response to an influx of calcium triggered by some external stimulus (Fig. 6). On the other hand, calpain-2 would be activated by a phosphorylation event as discussed before, and participates in disassembling the focal adhesion, which prevents cells from migrating. Thus, calpain-1 and calpain-2 are involved in a push-pull mechanism that allows cells to move.

The idea that evolution often does not seem to follow what we consider an intelligent design has been extensively developed by the French biologist Francois Jacob for whom evolution is just a blind tinkerer[9], which takes whatever is available in order to improve the way things work. In neurons, these mechanisms are used for regulating dendritic and spine formation as well as axonal elongation. In adult neurons, the same processes are used to regulate synaptic plasticity by controlling the machinery involved in determining the three-dimensional structure of the dendritic spines.

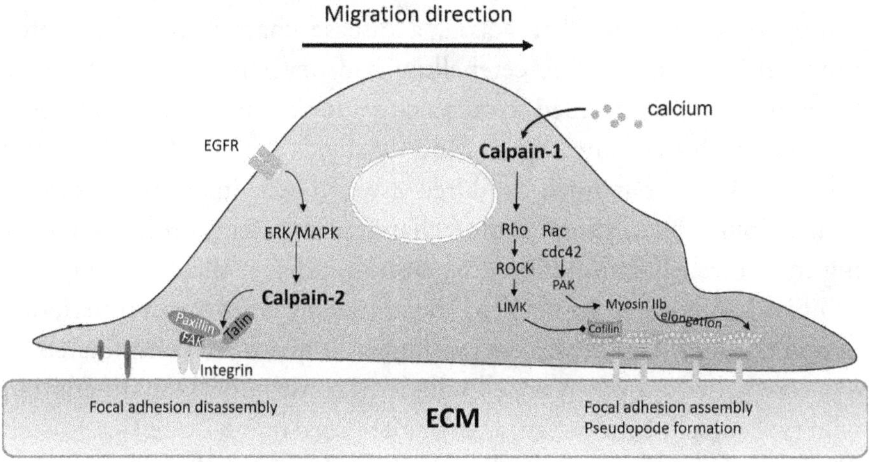

Figure 6: Schematic representation of the roles of calpain-1and calpain-2 in cell migration.

In our model, we postulate that calpain-1 is activated by an influx of calcium triggered by some external stimulus, resulting in the formation of pseudopods, which would elongate the cell and facilitate migration. On the other hand, calpain-2 would be activated by a phosphorylation event possibly triggered by the activation of the EGF receptor and results in the disassembly of the focal adhesion points maintaining the cell on its substrate (modified from Baudry and Bi, 2016[8]).

If calpain-1 and calpain-2 play opposite functions in synaptic plasticity, could it be that they also play opposite functions in neurodegeneration? Another talented postdoc, Dr. Yubin Wang, started to work on this question. It rapidly became apparent that this was indeed the case. In a series of very clever experiments, he showed that calpain-1 was part of a complex of synaptic proteins containing one subtype of the NMDA receptors, which had been shown to be neuroprotective, the NR2A receptors. Activation of this pathway led to the stimulation of a neuroprotective signaling cascade. In contrast, calpain-2 appeared to be associated with an extrasynaptic subtype of the NMDA receptors, the NR2B receptors, which had been shown to lead to the activation of a neurodegenerative signaling cascade[10].

Interestingly, after the publication of a manuscript reporting that calpain-1 was neuroprotective, I received an email from a British neurologist saying that he was following a patient with a mutation in calpain-1, which would result in a lack of enzymatic activity, and this patient exhibited severe cerebellar ataxia, a disease characterized by motor function impairment. The cerebellum had never been a structure we focused on, but we decided to take a closer look at our calpain-1 knock-out mice both anatomically and functionally. Indeed, we found that the calpain-1 knock-out mice exhibited a locomotor impairment similar to that found in the human cerebellar ataxia patient, probably resulting from cerebellar alterations. We also found that these mutant mice exhibited an increase in neuronal death during the postnatal period, a period during which the excessive number of neurons are eliminated by a process called apoptosis or cell suicide, as compared to the situation in wild type mice[11]. In addition, a particular breed of dogs, the Jack Russell Terrier, had also been reported to exhibit spino-cerebellar ataxia and to have a mutation in the calpain-1 gene[12]. Thus, in mouse, dog and human, a lack of function mutation in the calpain-1 gene or a deletion of the gene results in cerebellar ataxia, which is due to alterations in the normal postnatal developmental program controlling the survival or death of neurons, as well as the maturation of dendritic spines. The lack of calpain-1 resulted in enhanced neuronal death during the postnatal period as well as the lack of maturation of dendritic spines in multiple brain regions, including the hippocampus and the cerebellum.

We summarized our findings in a publication entitled "Calpain-1 and calpain-2: the yin and yang of synaptic plasticity and neurodegeneration"[13]. In this review, we argued that calpain-1 activation was required for triggering the molecular cascades leading to long-term potentiation and learning and memory and neuroprotection. On the other hand, a brief period of calpain-2 activation limits the extent of potentiation and of learning and memory. In addition, prolonged calpain-2 activation results in extensive neurodegeneration. It is important to realize that there are two different mechanisms for calpain-2 activation. One, which is short and reversible requires a phosphorylation event, which can be triggered by BDNF, and a low calcium concentration. This form of calpain-2 activation is responsible for the negative regulation of synaptic plasticity and learning and memory. The other one is prolonged and irreversible and requires phosphorylation and a high calcium concentration. This condition presumably leads to self-truncation of calpain-2, resulting in an unregulated state of activation, which will last for the life of the protein. This mechanism of activation is involved in the neurodegenerative function of calpain-2 and takes place in many different conditions, such as after a concussion, or after a seizure.

While we have focused our studies on acute forms of neurodegeneration, it is perfectly plausible that this mechanism also takes place in more chronic forms of neurodegeneration, such as in Parkinson's disease, Alzheimer's disease and ALS. As we mentioned before, I had received funding from the NIH to test the potential use of calpain inhibitors in animal models of Parkinson's disease, but did not reach any positive conclusions, since at that time, I did not realize that we needed to use selective calpain-2 inhibitors. It might well be worth it now to test selective calpain-2 inhibitors in animal models of PD and AD. I have now established a collaboration with Dr. Amy Arnsten at Yale University, and she will shortly start testing NA-184 in her animal model of AD. She has showed that old monkeys exhibit all the symptoms of the human disease, including neuronal death, amyloid plaques and neurofibrillary tangles. In addition, there is a strong rationale linking calpain-2 activation to the development of these pathological manifestations of the disease. As mentioned above, she has already shown that a selective calpain-2 inhibitor enhances learning in her aged monkeys.

Finally, we provided evidence that one of the mechanisms responsible for these opposite functions of calpain-1 and calpain-2 was their associations to different clusters of proteins, resulting in different subcellular localizations, with calpain-1 being localized synaptically downstream of the NMDA receptors, while calpain-2 was predominantly localized extrasynaptically and downstream of a different subtype of NMDA receptors (Fig. 7).

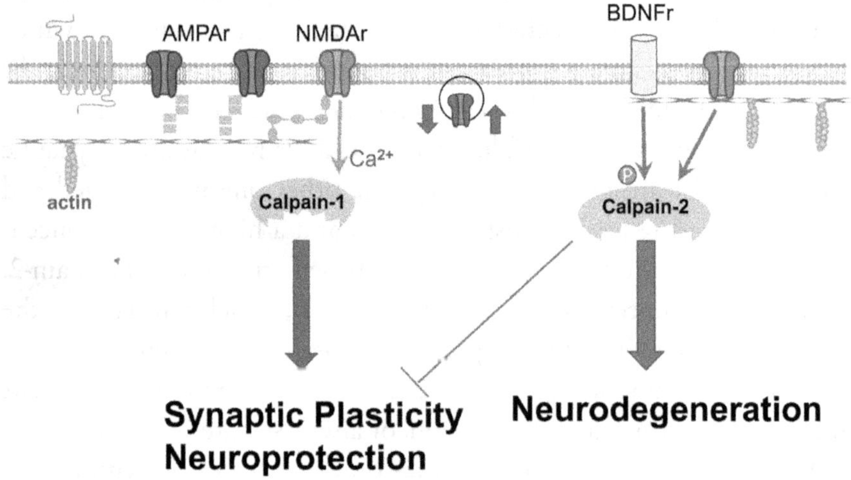

Figure 7: Opposite functions of calpain-1 and calpain-2 in the brain.

Calpain-1 is localized mostly in synapses downstream of the NMDA receptors and its activation results in synaptic plasticity and is neuroprotective. On the other hand, calpain-2 is localized extrasynaptically, and its activation limits the extent of synaptic plasticity and is neurodegenerative.

As mentioned several times in this book, science works in apparently unpredictable ways. Our brain is continuously analyzing information from internal and external sources and trying to make sense of all the data accumulated by years of experience. Indeed, some people are extremely good at this, and I was always in awe of some of my classmates at Ecole Polytechnique who could at the end of a complicated math lecture explain to me in great details what was discussed in the lecture and how it integrated with the whole field of mathematics. Clearly, I am much slower, and it takes me months and even years for integrating all the information I am accumulating. Consider that I started to work on calpain around 1979 and it took me almost 40 years to start figuring out what calpains were doing in the brain. As I kept telling my students, either I am very stupid, or the problem was complicated. I suppose it is probably a combination of both. Moreover, as scientists accumulate fundamental knowledge, they also face a growing desire to make concrete applications of this knowledge and to translate their discoveries into products that could be useful for humanity. I was not immune to this, as I had been exposed repeatedly to such desire, and this is what drove the directions of my next studies.

Chapter 11
STARTING TBI WORK

By 2016, it became clear that calpain-2 could indeed be an important target for acute neurodegeneration, and that selective calpain-2 inhibitors could have a broad range of clinical applications. As discussed in Chapter 1, this is when I decided to start NeurAegis, as I thought we would be able to move faster to develop such selective inhibitors for specific clinical applications. When we started NeurAegis in 2016, we had already identified a prototype selective calpain-2 inhibitor, C2I, aka NA-101, by examining the compounds that had been synthesized for Cortex Pharmaceuticals by Dr. Powers at Georgia Tech. We had tested this molecule on LTP in hippocampal slices and found that it did enhance the magnitude of LTP[1]. We had also found that it enhanced learning and memory in normal mice when administered before training[2]. As mentioned above, we also found that it restored normal learning and memory in the calpain-1 knock-out mice, suggesting that a selective calpain-2 inhibitor could be beneficial for disorders associated with learning and memory impairment. By that time, I really wanted to work on acute neurodegeneration, since from my previous experience I knew that working on models of chronic neurodegeneration was extremely difficult and that the animal models were not very predictive of what happens in humans. As mentioned above, we have cured Alzheimer's disease in mice close to 100 times, but nothing has translated to humans so far. I just happened to read a publication reporting results from an animal model of acute glaucoma, which looked relatively easy to implement. While there are various forms of glaucoma, acute glaucoma or more precisely acute angle-closure glaucoma, is associated with severe eye pain, nausea and vomiting and blurred vision. If not taken care of rapidly, it can lead to blindness. Western University of Health Sciences has a College of Optometry, and I knew a couple of the college faculty who were interested in glaucoma. With their help, we set up a mouse model of acute glaucoma, which consisted in increasing intraocular pressure to high levels by injecting a saline solution in the eye. This can be calibrated accurately by using the same tools your optometrist uses for determining your intraocular pressure. In our model, we increased intraocular pressure for one hour, after which pressure was returned to normal. In the days following this manipulation, a large number of retinal ganglion cells, the cells that are responsible for sending visual information to the brain, die and the animal becomes blind. This is in fact what happens in humans experiencing an acute glaucoma episode during which intraocular pressure rises rapidly and, if not taken care immediately, the person will indeed become blind.

Scientists have developed clever means to determine how much a mouse can see, and in collaboration with our colleagues from the College of Optometry, we implemented one of these tests in our laboratory. We showed that a single administration of C2I either systemically or intraocularly one hour after the return of intraocular pressure to normal completely prevented the death of retinal ganglion cells and the development of blindness. We also verified that this was associated with a complete prevention of calpain-2 activation in the eye[3]. These results gave us confidence that we were on the right track, and they confirmed that calpain-2 was indeed the right target to prevent acute neurodegeneration. In addition, we also verified in this model that the calpain-1 knock-out mice, which lack calpain-1 in retinal ganglion cells, were more susceptible than their wildtype strain to increased intraocular pressure, as they exhibited more neuronal death in the retina in this model of acute glaucoma, further validating our hypothesis that calpain-1 and calpain-2 were performing opposite functions in the brain.

However, acute angle-closure glaucoma is not very common in Western populations, although it is much more prevalent in Asian populations. Nevertheless, as my friend and co-founder of NeurAegis, Bernard, was at the time on the board of a biotech company in Boston developing technologies for eye disorders, we did initiate discussions to license our selective inhibitor for the treatment of eye disorders with this small biotech. However, these discussions did not lead to a licensing agreement, as the biotech company realized that it would not have the resources needed to pursue the clinical development of our selective calpain-2 inhibitor for the treatment of glaucoma. While I am still convinced that developing a selective calpain-2 inhibitor for the treatment of acute glaucoma would be extremely beneficial for a large patient population in Asia and throughout the World, I also concluded that this was not the first clinical indication that we wanted to pursue for the treatment of patients in the US and the Western World.

We turned our attention to traumatic brain injury for several reasons. First, and as we discussed above, it is very prevalent and the number of patients experiencing concussion/traumatic brain injury is very high. Second, there was then and there is still now not a single treatment targeting neuronal damage. Finally, several animal models have been developed for various types of concussion. We selected the model referred to as controlled cortical impact (Fig. 1). In this model, mice are anesthetized and placed in what is called a stereotactic apparatus. This means that the head is positioned very precisely, and we can select the localization of the impact in a reproducible manner. A small hole is drilled through the skull and a piston positioned to hit the surface of the brain at a specified speed and to a specified depth. This model has a number of advantages and in particular, it produces very reproducible brain lesions. Like what happens in a human suffering an open brain trauma, the initial impact results in a small lesion at the site of the impact, and the cells in this area die rapidly as a result of the impact. Moreover, in the days after the impact, the area surrounding the impact undergoes further neurodegeneration and the size of the lesion increases. This process takes many days, and this is the period of time when calpain-2 activation is critical for the death of these neurons.

Controlled Cortical Impact (CCI) model of TBI

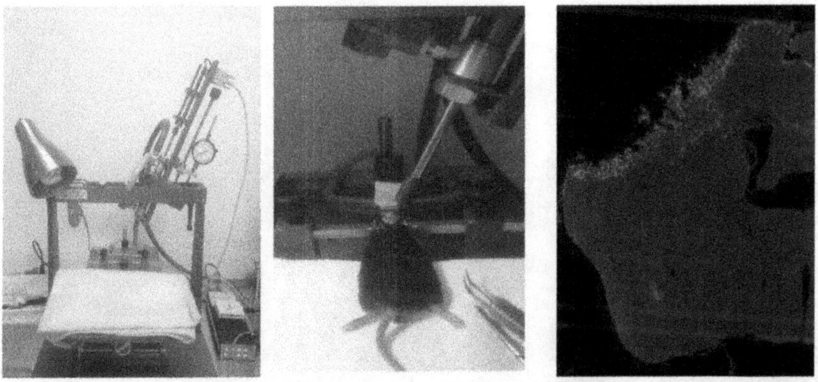

Figure 1: Mouse model of TBI

On the left is a picture of the device we used to develop the controlled cortical impact mouse model of TBI. This consists of a stereotaxic apparatus, which allows to precisely position the head of the mouse, a piston precisely controlled for speed and depth of penetration in the brain. Middle: mice are anesthetized and placed in the stereotaxic apparatus. A small incision is made in the skull to allow penetration of the piston to a depth of 3 mm. Right: brain section stained for degenerating cells.

This model replicates to some extent what takes place in a human experiencing an open skull accident (car accident, gunshot, hit on the head, etc.). However, because we could precisely control the location of the impact, the speed of the piston and the depth of penetration, the consequences of the trauma are very reproducible from one animal to the next, as opposed to human subjects experiencing open skull TBI. Importantly, we could measure multiple parameters in this model, including motor activity, learning performance in various tests of memory, the levels of calpain activation in the area surrounding the lesion, the number of dying neurons, as well as markers of brain inflammation. In our experiments, we started by administering NA-101 systemically 1 h after the trauma, and we analyzed several parameters related to the extent of the lesion, the extent of cell death, the degree of calpain-1 and calpain-2 activation, and the locomotor and cognitive impairments. One of the first observations we made was that mice treated with NA-101 appeared to have a much smaller brain lesion already 24 h after the trauma (Fig. 2).

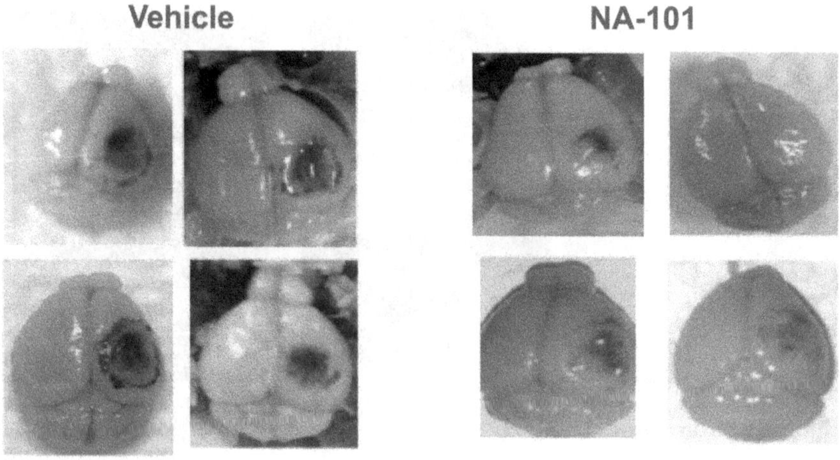

Figure 2: Effects of NA-101 on brain lesion 24 h after TBI.

Mice were subjected to TBI and received an injection of NA-101 1 h later. They were sacrificed 24 h later and the brains were extracted from the skull and photos were taken. As can be seen in the vehicle-treated mice, the impact resulted in a large lesion as well as significant blood infiltration. In contrast, animals receiving an injection of NA-101 had a much smaller lesion and much less blood infiltration.

A widely used task to analyze locomotor activity in rodents is called the beam walking task (Fig. 3). In this task, the mouse or the rat is placed on a wooden beam and the animal has to cross the beam to find a secure box on the other side of the beam. The time to cross and the number of foot slips are analyzed, as they represent quantitative measures of locomotor function. In the days following TBI, mice treated with vehicle were much slower to cross the beam and made many more foot slips than mice treated with NA-101[4].

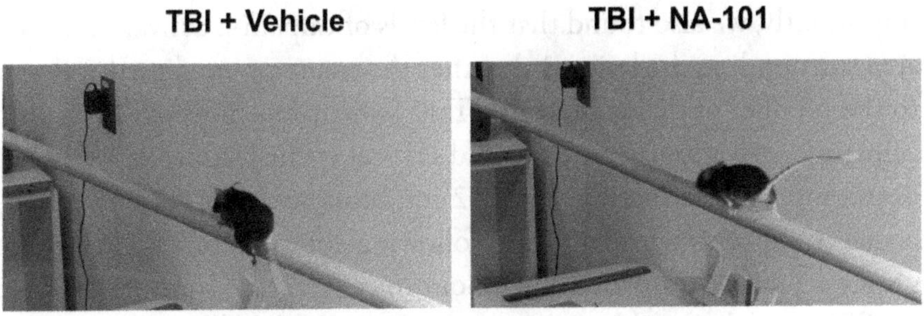

Figure 3: Beam walking after TBI.

On the left is a picture of a mouse 1 day after TBI and treated with the vehicle. The rear left paw is shown flipping from the beam. This mouse is also much slower to cross the beam than the mouse on the right, which has been treated with NA-101 1 h after TBI. The number of foot slips is also significantly reduced.

We also found smaller lesions in the days following the surgery and improved cognitive performance one week following surgery[4]. This model also allowed us to determine the time-course of activation of both calpain-1 and calpain-2 in the brain area surrounding the lesion. What we found was very surprising. Calpain-1 was rapidly but transiently activated, as if the brain first attempted to stimulate a neuroprotective pathway but failed to maintain it. On the other hand, calpain-2 activation was slightly delayed but remained elevated for days after the trauma (Fig. 4a). This was precisely what we had found in the glaucoma model (Fig. 4b).

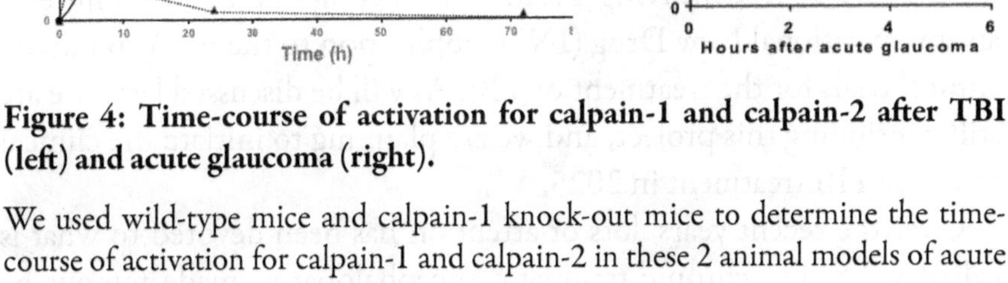

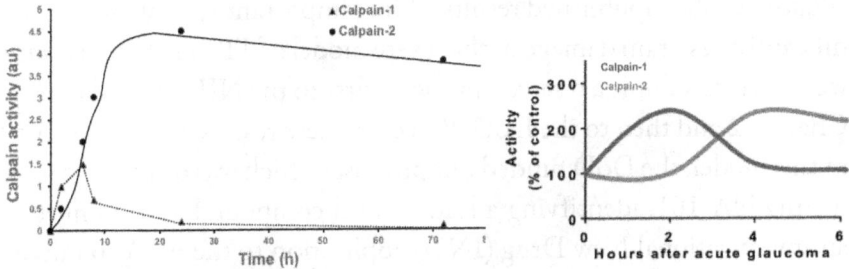

Figure 4: Time-course of activation for calpain-1 and calpain-2 after TBI (left) and acute glaucoma (right).

We used wild-type mice and calpain-1 knock-out mice to determine the time-course of activation for calpain-1 and calpain-2 in these 2 animal models of acute neurodegeneration.

Importantly, we also found that the levels of calpain-2 activation in the area surrounding the lesion 1 day after the trauma were directly related to the number of dying neurons[4]. This provided us more evidence that calpain-2 activation is an early and critical event leading to neuronal death and that a selective calpain-2 inhibitor could be extremely beneficial to prevent neuronal death following concussion/TBI. As in the glaucoma model, calpain-1 knock-out mice were also more susceptible to TBI than their wildtype strain, as the size of the brain lesion produced by the same trauma was larger in these mice[5]. To further validate the role of calpain-2 in this model, we decided to create what is called a conditional calpain-2 knock-out mouse. Unlike the global calpain-1 knock-out mice, which are lacking calpain-1 in every cell and organ but are perfectly viable and able to reproduce, global calpain-2 knock-out mice die during embryonic development, which indicates that calpain-2 plays a critical role during the embryonic period. This might also explain why such a potentially damaging enzyme has not been eliminated during evolution.

Scientists have developed technologies that enable the deletion of selective genes in selected cellular populations in order to bypass this type of problem. We therefore used one of these technologies to selectively delete calpain-2 in all the excitatory neurons of the forebrain[6]. These mice proved to be very interesting. As we had predicted, they exhibited enhanced learning abilities in two tests of learning we subjected them to (Baudry et al., unpublished results). More importantly, they showed significantly less brain damage in the severe model of TBI[7]. All these results were used to submit a research proposal first to the NIH, as discussed in Chapter 2 and then to the DoD. Based on these results we had obtained in this model, the DoD funded our proposal which was directed at optimizing NA-101, identifying a lead clinical compound and submitting an Investigational New Drug (IND) application to the FDA to initiate clinical trials for the treatment of TBI. As will be discussed later, we are still continuing this project, and we are planning to initiate the clinical trials for TBI treatment in 2025.

Over the recent years, lots of attention has been devoted to what is called CTE, i.e., chronic traumatic encephalopathy, made famous by the movie "Concussion", starring Will Smith. As discussed earlier, CTE was discovered in 2002 by Dr. Bennet Omalu when he performed the autopsy of the Pittsburgh Steelers center Mike Webster. This condition seems to be quite prevalent in NFL football players, and has revealed the problems associated with repeated concussions, even mild ones. CTE is characterized by massive accumulation of hyperphosphorylated tau, gliosis, and neurodegeneration. Several scientists think that hyperphosphorylated tau protein misfolds and acts like the famous prion protein discovered by the Nobel prize winner, Dr. Stanley Prusiner. In this hypothesis, misfolded tau would propagate in the brain and produce widespread neuronal damage and inflammation[8].

We therefore decided to investigate whether our selective calpain-2 inhibitor could also prevent the development of CTE, and we again used a mouse model for these studies. Mice were equipped with a small helmet and were subjected to repeated hits on the head several times a day and for several days (Fig. 4).

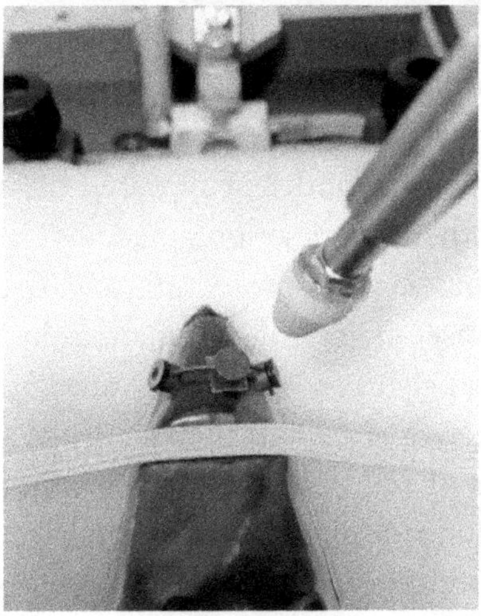

Figure 4: Mouse model of repeated mild TBI.

In this model, mice are temporally immobilized and are equipped with a helmet. They are subjected to repeated concussions several times a day and for 10 days.

These mice went on to develop a brain pathology very similar to what has been reported for human CTE patients, including brain inflammation, axonal injury and cognitive impairment. We implemented this model in our laboratory, and we decided to use mini-pumps to deliver NA-101 slowly and continuously during the whole period of repeated concussions. In fact, the pumps were implanted in the mice the day before the treatment and remained in place for 2 weeks. Mice treated with our selective calpain-2 inhibitor, NA-101, were completely protected against all these pathological manifestations. They showed no neuronal degeneration, no brain inflammation, no tau hyperphosphorylation and no cognitive impairment[8]. As mentioned earlier, we had mutant mice with selective deletion of calpain-2 in one category of neurons, the excitatory neurons of the forebrain, and we subjected these mice to the same protocol of repeated concussions for 10 days. After 1 month, these mice also showed no neuronal degeneration, no brain inflammation, no tau hyperphosphorylation and no cognitive impairment[9]. These results clearly showed that the effects we had seen with NA-101 treatment were due to the selective inhibition of calpain-2, and not to some other potential effects of the drug on a different target. They also showed that prolonged calpain-2 activation resulting from repeated concussions plays a critical role in the development of CTE.

It is worth stressing the significance of these results. Thus, in both a model of severe TBI as well as in a model of repeated mild TBI, down-regulating calpain-2 with either genetic or pharmacological intervention resulted in highly significant neuroprotection and the elimination of many pathological consequences of the trauma, including neuronal death and functional impairments. Moreover, our data indicating that levels of calpain-2 activation around the site of the impact were directly related to the levels of cell death strongly supported the idea that calpain-2 activation is indeed one of the critical events leading to neuronal damage. They also indicated that a selective calpain-2 inhibitor could efficiently protect the brain when administered shortly after the trauma and for a relatively short period of time, around 7 days. Thus, we had clearly identified a cellular mechanism that played a major role in the development of neuronal degeneration and the associated pathological manifestations of mild or severe concussion. We also had a prototype of a molecule that could inhibit this cellular process and be further developed for potential clinical applications.

Chapter 12
FINDING THE RIGHT MOLECULE

Throughout this book, I often referred to C2I as NA-101, since it was the first selective calpain-2 inhibitor that we had identified at WesternU, when we started NeurAegis. As we discussed, we have shown that it exerted neuroprotective effects in both acute glaucoma and in TBI in mice. However, this molecule had previously been patented by Cortex and therefore we could not patent it, although we could have tried to patent its use for treating concussion/TBI. This type of molecules, which are peptidomimetics have what chemists call chirality centers, which are atoms, generally carbon, with four different groups attached in a way that can create mirror images, also called stereoisomers[1]. C2I has 2 such chirality centers, which therefore generate two diastereoisomers, which are defined as R,S- and S,S-C2I. In biochemistry the S-form of amino acids is the dominant and active form, as opposed to its mirror image, the R-form. Using an in vitro assay for calpain-2 activity, we first confirmed that S,S-C2I was the active form, and that R,S-C2I had no inhibitory activity. We therefore tried to patent this form of C2I as our first patent application, arguing that the previous patent from Cortex, which reported this molecule, was only referring to the mixture of the two forms, the R,S and the S,S. However, the patent examiner rejected our claim of novelty and instead concluded that the molecule had previously been described as a calpain inhibitor.

We then decided that we needed to make novel analogs of this molecule with better drug-like features, which we could then patent as novel chemical entities (NCE). Thanks to one of NeurAegis's scientific advisors, Dr. Philippe Bey, we found a medicinal chemistry Contract Research Organization (CRO), Nanosyn, which was willing to start working on synthesizing analogs of this molecule and to defer payment until NeurAegis could raise the financing needed for drug development. In parallel, I submitted multiple grant applications to federal agencies to support the development program. As discussed above, after several unsuccessful attempts with the NIH, these efforts were successful, and we received funding from the CDRMP to identify a novel selective calpain-2 inhibitor suitable for clinical trials. Having funding to synthesize analogs led to intense and productive discussions between chemists and biologists to design new molecules, to synthesize them and to test them in our lab.

There are generally two ways to identify novel molecules targeting a specific protein. The first one is called high-throughput screening, in which thousands of molecules are tested using an assay compatible for such an approach. While we did have such an assay, which consists in incubating the molecules with purified calpain-1 or calpain-2 and a fluorescent substrate and evaluating the changes in fluorescence following cleavage of the substrate, we did not have either access to these thousands of molecules, nor the robotic equipment needed to perform these kinds of experiments. This is what the pharmaceutical industry generally does, since it has both the libraries of molecules and the equipment.

The other approach is called medicinal chemistry and involves refining existing molecules to generate, through organic chemistry, new molecules, which could become drug-like agents. We started working with a very talented computational chemist, Dr. Lyna Luo, at the College of Pharmacy at WesternU, and she used what is called docking to place C2I in the 3-dimension model of calpain-2. She indeed verified that the S-S isomer was able to fit much better in the active site of calpain-2 than the S,R isomer (Fig. 1). She also showed that the chemical groups on both sides of the C2I molecule were critical to determine the specificity of these molecules for calpain-1 or calpain-2[2]. This information was then used to design the first C2I analogs, which were synthesized by Nanosyn. These analogs were then tested in in vitro and in vivo assays for calpain-1 and calpain-2. Results obtained with this initial batch of molecules were then used to redesign new analogs and the cycle continued until we selected some lead compounds to be tested in the in vivo TBI model (Fig.2).

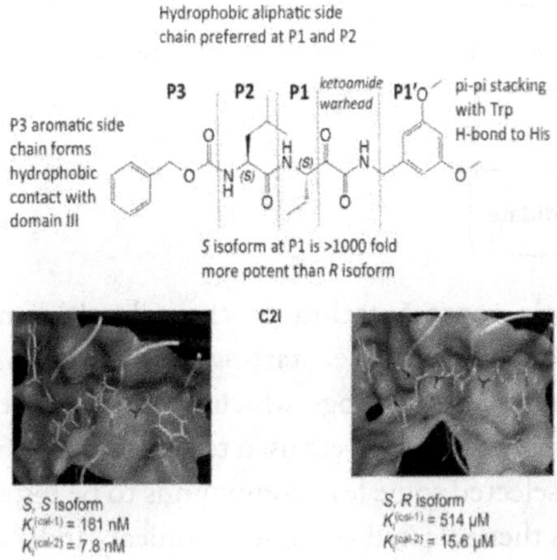

Figure 1: Chemical structure of C2I (NA-101) and docking of its 2 diastereoisomers in the active site of calpain-2.

C2I is a peptidomimetic with 2 chiral centers (S), which binds to a cysteine amino acid in calpain-2. Bottom left represents the binding of the S,S isoform, and bottom right the binding of the S,R isoform. (From Figure 3 of Baudry et al., 2023, Neurotherapeutics, https://doi.org/10.1007/s13311-023-01407-y, Copyright Elsevier).

The new molecules were first tested in in vitro assays for calpain-1 and calpain-2 activity. In these assays, purified enzymes from various sources (mostly human and porcine) were incubated with a fluorescence substrate, which, once cleaved by calpain, produces a molecule with different fluorescent properties than the initial substrate. Adding various concentrations of the putative inhibitors led to the determination of the selectivity (calpain-2 versus calpain-1) and the potency (how much of the inhibitor is needed to completely block calpain activity) of the various molecules[3]. Results from these experiments were then used to

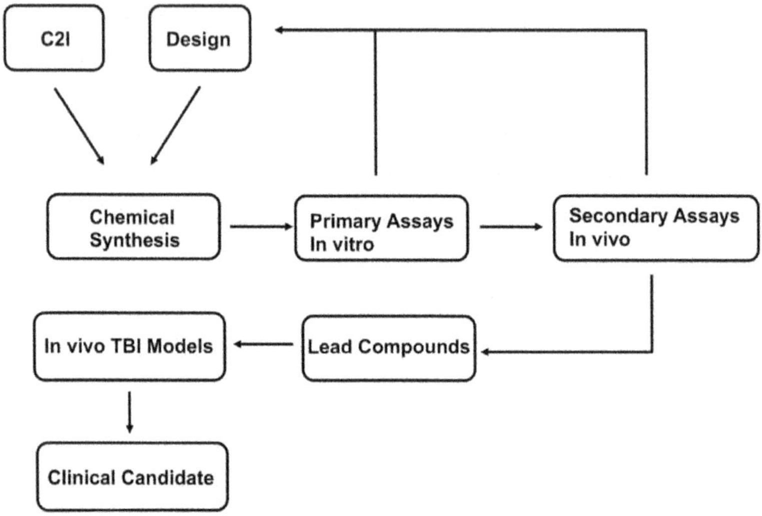

Figure 2: Schematic representation of the selection method we used to identify the lead clinical candidate. Starting from the initial calpain-2 inhibitor, C2I, we designed a number of analogs, which were synthesized and then tested in in vitro and in vivo assays. Results were used to redesign new analogs and the cycle continued until we selected some lead compounds to be tested in the in vivo TBI model. NA-184 was then selected as our lead clinical candidate.

design new inhibitors with better selectivity and potency. These primary in vitro assays were followed by secondary assays in which the molecules were tested for their inhibitory activity against mouse brain calpain-1 and calpain-2 (Fig. 3). We used two tools to perform these experiments. The first tool was the key difference between calpain-1 and calpain-2, which is their calcium sensitivity. Calpain-1 requires low concentrations of calcium for activation, and thus, we used 20 μM calcium in the assay for calpain-1 and 2,000 μM for calpain-2. However, this high calcium concentration activates both calpain-1 and calpain-2. Our second tool was the calpain-1 knock-out mouse. As we discussed previously, these mice have been engineered by Dr. Athar Chishti at Tufts University and lack calpain-1 globally but have normal calpain-2 levels. Therefore, by using brain homogenates from these calpain-1 knock-out (KO) mice we could selectively test the potency of the newly synthesized molecules against calpain-2.

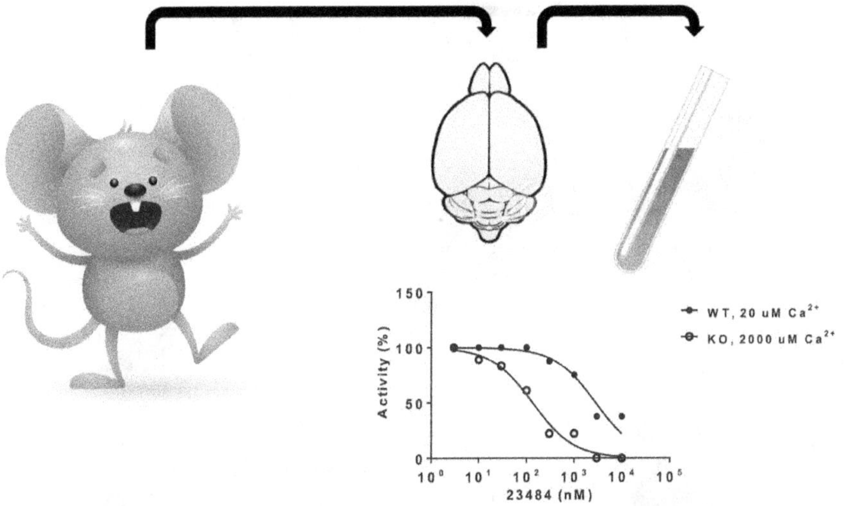

Figure 3: Testing selective calpain-2 inhibitors against mouse brain calpain-1 and calpain-2. Brains from wild-type or calpain-1 knock-out mice were dissected and homogenized. Calpain-1 and calpain-2 activity were assayed in the homogenates in the presence of various concentrations of the inhibitors.

This was followed by the in vivo testing of the best molecules identified by the in vitro assays. We had an additional tool to determine the in vivo selectivity of the newly synthesized molecules for calpain-1 or calpain-2. Due to their chemical nature, the newly synthesized molecules make a reversible covalent bond with calpain-1 or calpain-2. This means that the molecules can bind to the enzyme and remain bound for a significant period of time. Because this bond is however reversible, the molecule will slowly unbind from the enzyme and the enzyme will exhibit full enzymatic activity. We could thus inject these molecules into the mice and take their brains at various times after injection and measured calpain-1 and calpain-2 activity in brain homogenates (Fig.4).

After synthesizing over 130 molecules, testing all of them in the *in vitro* models, and a large number in the in vivo models, we had a short list of 5-6 molecules with a much better in vivo selectivity for calpain-2 than calpain-1. We then tested them in the controlled cortical impact model of TBI, by injecting these inhibitors 1 h after the trauma. Various parameters were then measured at various times after the trauma. In particular, we measured calpain-1 and calpain-2 activity in brain

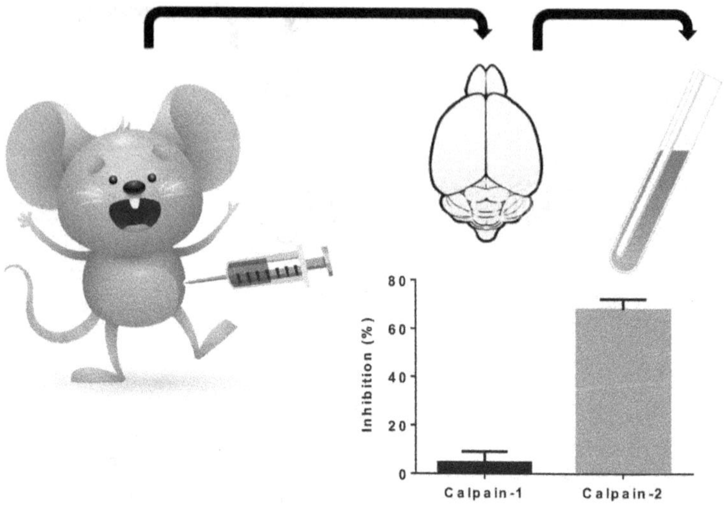

Figure 4: In vivo assay for calpain selectivity of newly synthesized calpain inhibitors.

In this example, NA-184 was injected intravenously (2 mg/kg) and mice sacrificed 30 min later. Their brains were dissected, and calpain-1 and calpain-2 activity were measured in brain homogenates. NA-184 showed a high selectivity for calpain-2 as there was almost no inhibition of calpain-1 compared to a 70% inhibition of calpain-1.

homogenates 24 h after the trauma. We discovered that a few inhibitors which were quite potent in the in vitro tests had no effect on either brain calpain-1 or calpain-2 activity. In parallel, they also did not have any neuroprotective activity. For us the logical conclusion was that these molecules could not cross the blood-brain barrier, this cellular complex we discussed earlier in Chapter 2. This is not uncommon for many molecules, which for one reason or another do not have the right features to move across the cellular membranes that make the blood-brain barrier.

We ended up focusing our efforts on two inhibitors, which we named NA-112 and NA-184, as these two molecules showed a high degree of selectivity for calpain-2 over calpain-1 and had a very significant neuroprotection effect in the mouse model of TBI. To be precise, NA-112 was synthesized before NA-184 and we did perform a number of experiments and tests with NA-112, as for a while we thought we were going to select NA-112 as our lead clinical molecule. NA-184 was synthesized a few months later and we discovered that it had a better profile than NA-112 in the TBI model. Considering all the properties of these molecules, we have now selected NA-184 as our lead clinical candidate. This took us more than 2 years, as the chemists could only synthesize 6-8 new molecules per month, and we then rushed to test these molecules in the various assays.

An important issue in biological research, which has been emphasized over the last 10-15 years, is the issue of sex. For too long, experimental biologists were performing their experiments only in males. One of the major reasons for this was to avoid the difficulties associated with the female sex cycle, which impacts many biological processes. For most scientists, the choice of using males for their experiments was intended to reduce the number of animals needed for their experiments, since performing the experiments at each stage of the cycle would indeed considerably increase the number of animals and the costs of the experiments. Nowadays, the NIH and all the Federal Agencies require the investigators to consider sex as a critical variable and to incorporate this parameter in the design of the experiments. This is even more important for TBI since recent studies have indicated that sport concussions are worse for women than for men[4]. While there could be several reasons for this, the critical point was that we needed to determine whether our selective calpain-2 inhibitors would be as effective to protect the brain after concussion in females as in males. It turned out to be true and for both NA-112 and NA-184, as we found similar degree of calpain-2 inhibition and of neuroprotection in male and female mice and male and female rats after TBI[5].

This result was a highly significant milestone, and we decided to terminate the program of synthesizing new molecules and to focus on the development of NA-184, i.e., to perform all the studies required to bring a molecule to the clinic, which are called the pre-clinical studies. All these results have recently been published (Baudry et al., 2024).

Chapter 13
DEVELOPING NA-184 FOR CLINICAL STUDIES

For an academic scientist, the process involved in bringing a molecule from the bench to the bedside seems quite straightforward. After all, in academia, we are accustomed to purchasing research molecules and drugs from a variety of commercial sources; we then search the scientific literature to find the appropriate dose to use in our experimental animals, and we inject the drugs and analyze their effects in our experimental paradigms. Obviously, the process is much more complicated when one is trying to develop a novel molecule to use for a human indication. The path is highly regulated, and one has to follow the rules set up by the Food and Drug Administration (FDA), which has very strict requirements before a new molecule can be administered in humans for any indication[1].

First, one needs to be able to synthesize large amounts of the molecule to be able to perform all the studies that are required by the FDA, which are called the pre-Investigational New Drug (IND) studies. In the initial phase, we only needed a few milligrams of each new molecule in order to test them in the in vitro and even in the in vivo models, since these drugs were quite potent, and we only administered very low doses in the animals. As you may remember, we were using doses not higher than 1 mg/kg. Considering that the average weight of a mouse is about 30 g, this means that we were using 0.03 mg/mouse. Because pre-IND studies include safety/toxicity studies, in which the highest possible dose needs to be administered to two animal species (usually rats and dogs), we needed grams and even 100s of grams of the molecule. Once the molecule starts to be administered in humans, kilograms of the drug will need to be manufactured. The scale-up of the synthesis for NA-184 from synthesizing a few milligrams to 100s of grams, turned out to be more challenging than we thought, and it took the chemists at Nanosyn several months to find a synthesis path that could indeed provide large amounts of NA-184 in a minimum number of steps for the synthesis. They ended up synthesizing the molecules using 8 different steps. The purity of the molecule is another critical parameter, as the FDA will not allow the development of a molecule that has some impurities at levels above 1%. The Nanosyn chemists succeeded in producing large amounts of NA-184 with more than 99% purity, which was another significant milestone.

The next problem was to decide which diastereoisomer we were going to develop. As discussed above, all our selective calpain-2 inhibitors have two chirality centers, and could thus exist in 2 different variants, the R,S and the S,S variants. This was also the case for NA-184. While we knew that the S,S variant was the active molecule, we also discovered, using our calpain assay, that the two variants rapidly interconvert in aqueous solution. Thus, within minutes in solution, the R,S inactive variant becomes the S,S active variant and conversely, the active S,S becomes the inactive R,S variant. This phenomenon is called epimerization and is quite common for many molecules with chirality centers. We therefore decided that there was no good reason to develop the active S,S-NA-184, and that we could develop the mixture of the 2 variants, which was generated by the synthetic schema developed by Nanosyn[2]. At least, we got a break here, since it would have been even more challenging to synthesize the active variant of NA-184.

Another important issue is the stability of the molecule, as this is a critical parameter for determining which storage conditions are optimal.

Clearly, nobody wants to develop a molecule which falls apart within days after its synthesis. We thus tested the stability of NA-184 under different conditions, such as -20 °C, 0-5 °C and room temperature. We were quite fortunate that NA-184 appears to be very stable under all these conditions at least up to 6 months.

In order to use the drug for clinical trials, the molecule must be manufactured in a specific way called Good Manufacturing Practice (GMP), which means that the drug is consistently produced in high quality and purity from batch to batch, is free of contamination, and that all the steps are reproducible and well documented[3]. While Nanosyn knows how to do this, we have not done it yet, since this step is required only once we start human clinical studies. At the current stage of pre-IND studies, we only need to use what is called Good Laboratory Practice (GLP) conditions to prepare the drug and to administer it to animals for the safety/toxicity studies. This was performed by Nanosyn and by the CROs we used for all our preclinical studies.

Another critical step for performing the pre-IND studies as well as for the clinical trial, is the identification of a suitable formulation. In the case of NA-184, this turned out to be a major problem. NA-184 is very poorly soluble in aqueous solutions. This has never been a problem for our animal experimentation, as we performed a lot of our in vitro experiments by solubilizing the molecules in dimethylsulfoxide (DMSO), a very commonly used solvent for difficult to solubilize molecules. Since we had decided to develop NA-184 for the treatment of TBI, it was clear from the outset that we will have to administer NA-184 by intravenous injection, as some of the patients might be unconscious at the time we would need to initiate treatment and could not be treated by any other modality. We had shown in our animal experimentation that intravenous delivery of NA-184 provided a similar degree of calpain-2 inhibition and neuronal protection as systemic injection or subcutaneous injection. Already when we started our experiments in the animals, we realized that DMSO was not the ideal solvent, since by itself it has significant pharmacological effects, and we needed to identify other formulations[4]. We succeeded in identifying two formulations, which provided a similar degree of calpain-2 inhibition and neuronal protection. One was by using a molecule called cyclodextrin, which is a polymer, which encapsulates the molecule and therefore allows it to remain in aqueous solutions[5]. The other one, which was suggested by one of my colleagues from the College of Pharmacy at WesternU consisted of an aqueous solution of phospholipids. Phospholipids are the major constituents of cell membranes and form micelles, which can also encapsulate the molecule and carry it through the blood stream to the brain. Phospholipids are indeed quite commonly used for the formulation of many drugs marketed for various human indications[6]. However, these formulations provided for solutions of NA-184 with a maximum concentration of at best 1 mg/ml.

As we mentioned above, the FDA requires to test the safety/toxicity of new molecules at the highest possible concentrations, and in two animal species. Any drug will produce toxic effects of some kind, if administered at a large enough dose. The key is to find what doses are safe and whether there is a sufficient "therapeutic window" of doses between levels that produce beneficial effects and levels that produce toxic effects. We were therefore trying to find a formulation providing for a concentration of NA-184 of 50 mg/ml. We did hire a CRO specializing in formulation with the goal of finding a suitable formulation for intravenous injection of 50 mg/ml of NA-184. Since most animal studies using intravenous injection consider an appropriate volume to be 1 ml/kg, this meant that we could administer a dose of 50 mg/kg. This would represent 50 times the dose of NA-184 that we found maximally effective in our rodent studies, and we were confident that the FDA would be satisfied by using such a dose for the safety/toxicity studies. While the CRO did identify a formulation allowing us to administer 50 mg/kg in the pre-IND studies, this formulation was not tolerated by dogs. While rats tolerated a single injection of this formulation, they also started showing negative reactions when we repeated the injections 5 times. We had to terminate all the in vivo studies with this formulation. We are now back to square one and need to find another suitable formulation. Luckily, many new drugs that are being developed are like ours, very insoluble in water and new technologies are being used to allow the delivery of these molecules. So, we are confident that we will find an appropriate formulation in the coming months and will be able to complete the pre-IND studies by the end of the year.

The typical development timelines for the pre-IND activities are shown in Table I. This is supposed to be done in 24 weeks. But we rapidly discovered that this is a very optimistic timeline. Lots of things can go wrong, and, as we discussed, in our case, several things went wrong.

Activity	0	1	2	3	4	5	6	7	8	9	10	11	12	13	14	15	16	17	18	19	20	21	22	23	24
Development and validation																									
Analysis and validation																									
Reporting and audit																									
General Toxicology																									
Range finding rodent/dog																									
28-day study Rodent/dog																									
Reporting and audit																									
Genetic Toxicology																									
Ames test																									
Chromosomal aberrations																									
Rodent in vivo micronucleus																									
Reporting and audit																									
Safety Pharmacology																									
hERG channel test																									
Cardiovascular Dog study																									
Respiratory Rodent study																									
CNS safety pharmacology in rats																									
Reporting and audit																									

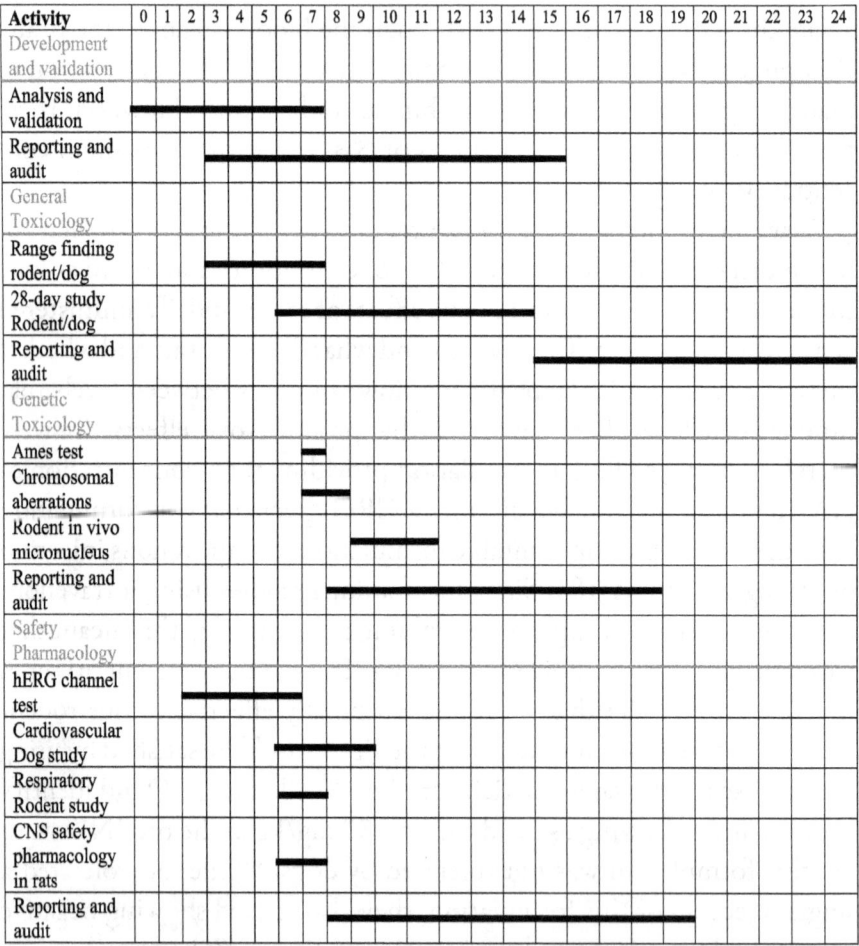

Table 1: Typical development timelines for pre-IND activities.
(modified from [7]).

The various activities, which are required by the FDA, in order to submit an Investigational New Drug (IND) application are outlined.

Moreover, when we started these activities in early 2021, we were still in the middle of the COVID epidemic. This resulted in many setbacks.

We found out the hard way that COVID had resulted in a huge increase in costs and long delays for all activities related to drug development, because so many new treatments and vaccines for Covid were being developed at the same time, leading to a shortage of manpower, supplies, and most importantly dogs, resulting in a huge increase in costs.

We quickly realized that we would not have enough funds in the budget provided by the CDRMP to cover the cost for all these activities. I communicated with the Program Officer in charge of our program, and the DoD agreed to provide a supplement to help us cover the additional costs, for which we are extremely grateful.

We are still on track to complete the pre-IND studies by end of 2024 and to submit our IND application to the FDA early 2025. This would still get us the possibility of starting a Phase I clinical trial for the treatment of TBI in 2025. This means that I will finally reach my long-term goal of giving a selective calpain-2 inhibitor to a human subject. At this point, this goal seems both so close and so far.

As I look back at the beginning of my journey more than 45 years ago, I am both humbled and grateful. I am humbled because I realize that it took so many people working not only in my lab but all over the World to get me to this point. While it is true that the number of people working on calpains is small, it still represents a significant number of scientists, who have dedicated their entire lives to understanding what these enzymes are doing in living organisms.

It is interesting to analyze the number of manuscripts that have been published since the identification of calpain in 1964 (Fig. 1).

While the calcium-dependent protease calpain was identified in 1964, it was not until the 1980s that Murachi renamed it calpain, which explains the lack of publications until 1980, which is the year I started publishing my first paper on calpains. The total number of publications as of May 2023 is 10,491. This is in fact a very small number of publications. If one uses neurodegeneration, PubMed lists more than 95,000 publications, and if one uses cancer, the number is over 4.7 million. With my more than 70 publications with calpain in the title, I have contributed almost 1% of the publications in the field. The field of calpain has a meeting every 3 years, which is directed at bringing together scientists from all over the World working on the roles of calpains in health and

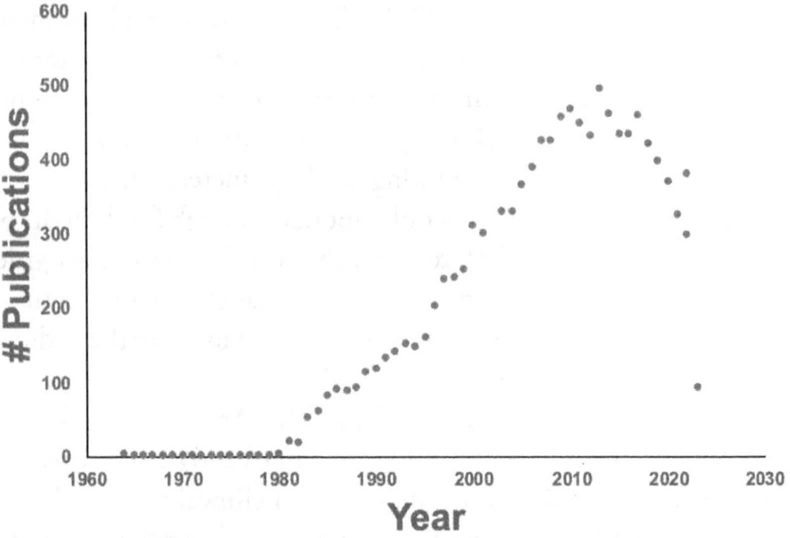

Figure 1: Number of publications on calpains per year since 1964.

These numbers are obtained from PubMed, a database from the NIH, which stores the majority of publications. It was searched using the keyword calpain.

diseases, and the 2022 meeting took place in Lisbon, Portugal. At this meeting, I received the Hiro Sumirachi lifetime achievement award, an award in honor of Hiro Sumirachi who made significant contributions to the field and unfortunately passed away in 2018.

I am grateful to all people who have helped me reaching this milesone, all the undergraduate and graduate students, as well as the postdocs who worked in my labs at UCI, USC and WesternU. They are the ones who ran most of the experiments I discussed in this book and who provided the evidence that a selective calpain-2 inhibitor could become a therapeutic treatment for TBI. I also feel like the runner of a marathon reaching the last mile of the race, both exhausted and exhilarated, as he/she could almost visualize the finish line. But of course, many people have said that the last mile is the most difficult one.

Chapter 14
CLINICAL TRIALS AND EXPECTATIONS

So, here we are, we can see the light at the end of the tunnel. As my mentor and friend Gary Lynch puts it, we are getting ready to "have a shot on goal." We are on the verge of achieving the dream of many scientists: seeing a lifelong career in academic research translated into tangible health benefits to patients who urgently need them. But, as Gary also points out, not many scientists get the chance to have a shot on goal.

Now is the time to plan for testing NA-184 in humans. Ahead of us are the Phase I, Phase II and Phase III clinical trials, the various steps required by the FDA before it will issue a New Drug Application (NDA) approval for sale and marketing of a new drug (Fig. 1).

The probability for developing new drugs, particularly "first in class" drugs like NA-184, has historically been low. A recent study from MIT indicates that approximately 2 percent of drugs in clinical trials eventually win approval from the FDA. However, several studies have shown that the availability of blood or other types of biomarkers very significantly improves the success rate of clinical trials up to 11% (Fig. 2)[2].

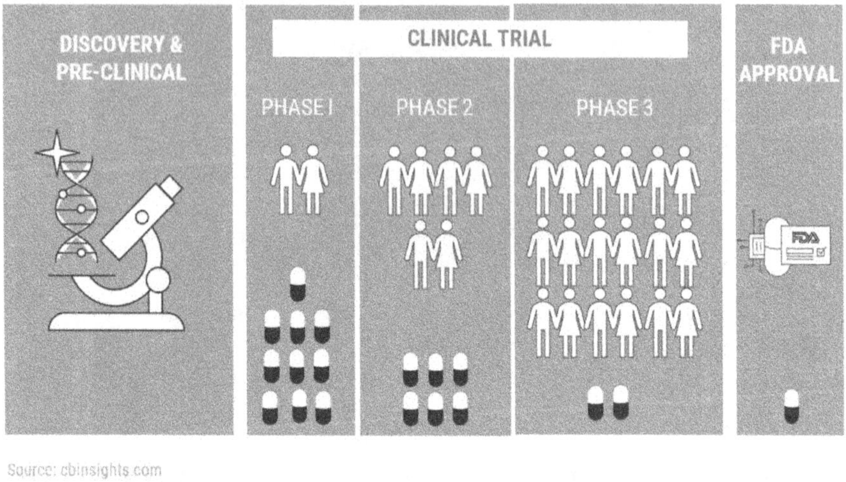

Figure 1: Typical path for moving a drug from pre-clinical to clinical and to FDA approval. From cbinsights.com[1]

Following the discovery and pre-clinical studies, clinical trials consist of 3 phases. Phase 1 tests the safety of the drug, generally in healthy subjects. Phase 2 tests its efficacy in a small sample of patients affected with the targeted disease. Phase 3 expands the Phase 2 to a much larger sample of patients from multiple centers and determine potential drug interaction. Each stage is accompanied by an attrition of the drugs moving from one phase to the next.

We are very fortunate to have such blood biomarkers for TBI. In fact, there are three blood biomarkers available for TBI. The first one is the protein Neurofilament light chain, or Nfl, which has now been shown to be a marker of axonal degeneration and leaks into the blood[3]. While this is not specific for TBI, any interference with axonal degeneration is expected to decrease blood levels of Nfl. In addition, there are two other blood biomarkers that are directly related to brain calpain-2 activation. The first one was discovered by Robert Siman at UPenn and represents a fragment of the neuronal protein we discussed earlier and that is cleaved by calpain, the cytoskeletal protein, spectrin, which has been named SNTF (Spectrin N-terminal Fragment). The reader may remember that we extensively used this cleavage in our animal experiments to analyze in vivo brain calpain activation. The UPenn group has shown that blood

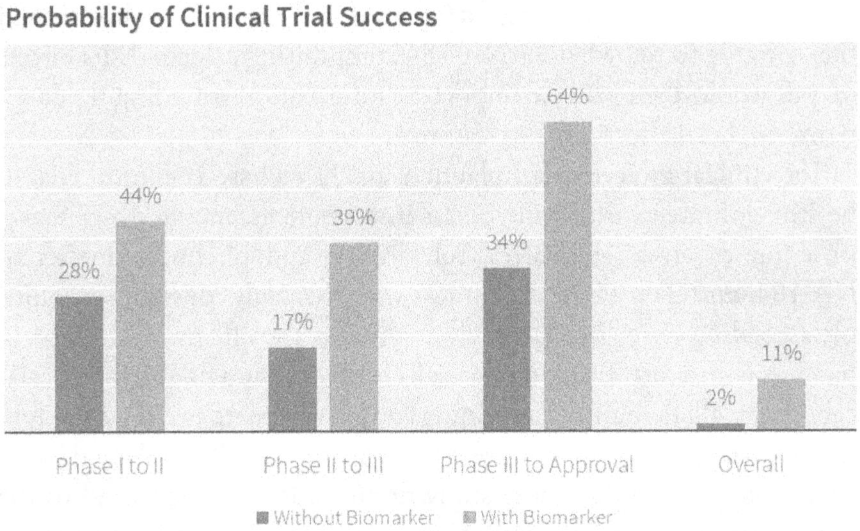

Figure 2: Probability of success for clinical trials for trials without a biomarker and for trials with a biomarker. (Source Nordvang, 2020[2])

levels of SNTF are elevated in the days following TBI and are predictive of the long-term consequences of TBI[4].

Importantly, our laboratory has identified another protein that is selectively cleaved by calpain-2 following TBI. It is a tyrosine protein phosphatase, that is a protein which removes a phosphate group from a tyrosine amino acid and is called PTPN13. Following cleavage by calpain-2, a fragment leaks into the blood, where we can measure it using an immunoassay. We have called this fragment P13BP and have shown that it is elevated in the blood in the days following TBI in both the mouse and rat models of TBI. In collaboration with a team of neurosurgeons at Arrowhead Regional Medical Center, a trauma center located within 20 miles of WesternU, we were able to show that P13BP levels were also elevated in the blood of human subjects 24 h after they experienced TBI. Furthermore, the levels of P13BP were correlated with the severity of the trauma, as measured with the Glasgow Coma Scale we discussed in Chapter 2[5].

Using these 3 blood biomarkers should provide important information regarding the ability of NA-184 to inhibit calpain-2 in the days after TBI in human subjects. Based on our animal experiments, we are planning to treat TBI patients for 7 days after the trauma, and we should then be able to tell whether NA-184 is inhibiting calpain-2. Its effects on Nfl would then provide important information regarding the long-term beneficial effects of the treatment.

The clinical interventions planned, are 1) a Phase Ia clinical trial in healthy volunteers that will consist in a single ascending dose (SAD) injection to assess the safety, tolerability, and pharmacokinetics of NA-184, and 2) a Phase Ib clinical trial that will consist in a multiple ascending dose (MAD) study evaluating the effects of NA-184 in patients with acute TBI. The Phase Ib study will be a double-blind, placebo-controlled, multiple ascending study to evaluate two dose levels in hospitalized patients with acute TBI. Dose levels will be selected based on the single ascending dose study findings. Patients admitted to the trauma center who meet entrance criteria will receive their first dose of study drug within 24 hours of documented TBI. Patients will receive twice daily dosing for 5 consecutive days. Study medication will be administered as an i.v. infusion over 20 minutes followed by collection of safety, tolerability, pharmacokinetic data.

After 40 + years of basic academic research in my and my wife's labs (we call ourselves "The Busy Bs"), we are finally on the verge of developing a new treatment for a devastating condition through NeurAegis. We plan to continue to work and to make further significant contributions to the field of neuroscience, which could also be commercialized through NeurAegis. My wife is particularly interested in understanding neurodevelopmental disorders, such as the Angelman Syndrome, a rare disease affecting about 50,000 children. I now also want to see, through NeurAegis, whether our selective calpain-2 inhibitors could be useful to treat other neurodegenerative diseases, such as epilepsy, loud noise-induced hearing loss and Alzheimer's disease. The next five years should be quite exciting.

Chapter 15
LESSONS LEARNED

It has been almost 45 years since I arrived at UC Irvine to start my postdoctoral fellowship. I came with my French wife and rapidly discovered that we were not a good fit, with me wanting to work in the lab all the time and her wanting to enjoy life in California. She went back to France, and we divorced shortly after. I embraced with passion the model that Gary Lynch had established in his lab where everybody was working hard, convinced that we were always on the verge of making breakthrough discoveries. This feeling became more acute after a few years when I became an Assistant Professor with my own lab and my own grants. I like the analogy between a lab director and an orchestra director, which has been made many times. For an orchestra to make great music, you not only need a great director but also great musicians. The same is true for the lab; you also need great scientists to make great science. I always thought of myself as the first violin in Gary's orchestra, and I tried to work with all the other postdocs and students to make sure we were doing great science. I have maintained the same approach even since, and I think I have succeeded over my 45 years of lab work to do great science. As Malcom Gladwell proposed[1], I believe in the 10,000-hour rule, which states that the key to achieve true expertise in any endeavor is simply a matter of dedicating 10,000 hours to that endeavor.

What did I learn during these 45 years of research? As discussed many times, to succeed in science one needs to be perseverant and be able to get up after falling and to keep going. In fact, many great scientists are afflicted with obsessive compulsive disorder[2], and it is probably true that many scientists are just obsessed with their work. I must admit that since I started working on calpains, I have been obsessed with trying to understand what their functions were, at least in the brain. As I discussed throughout this book, I think that we now know in much greater detail what capain-1 and calpain-2 are doing. To make it simple, it looks like calpain-1 is the "good" enzyme. It helps neurons to mature and to survive during the postnatal period and in the adult, it keeps the neurons alive and is critical for certain types of learning, and in particular, for what we have discussed as episodic learning, the ability to store daily events of our lives. As a result, loss of function mutations or lack of calpain-1 are associated with lack of maturation of neurons, excessive neuronal loss during the developmental period, learning impairment, and excessive damage following any insults of injuries. An agent able to selectively facilitate calpain-1 activation could be extremely beneficial as it would stimulate learning and neuroprotection. On the other hand, an inhibitor of calpain-1 would be detrimental for many brain functions. As we discussed in the previous chapters, this is probably the reason why the previous attempts to develop non-selective calpain inhibitors did not show significant beneficial effects.

In contrast, calpain-2 is the "bad" enzyme. It limits the amount of learning, at least for episodic learning, and it triggers neuronal damage after any insult or injury. It could also play an important role during the aging process and participate in progressive neuronal damage in chronic neurodegenerative disorders. As we discussed extensively, a selective calpain-2 inhibitor could not only facilitate learning but also represent an effective neuroprotective agent. We will know shortly whether these predictions are true, since we will be testing such a molecule in humans starting in 2024.

Scientists always want to discover general principles from the studies of selected examples. This is the basis of inductive reasoning where one goes from specific observations to general principles. Thus, it is reasonable to ask whether these findings regarding the functions of calpain-1 and calpain-2 in the brain also apply for other systems. We already discussed that what we found in the brain also applied to the eye, which is not surprising since after all, the eye is part of the brain. But what of other systems, like the heart or the kidney or the lungs? Unfortunately, there is not a lot of literature discussing this question, a point which has always astonished me. This question is also more difficult to answer since we now know that there are actually 15 members in the calpain family, from calpain-1 to calpain-16 (it turns out that calpain-4 is actually a small form of calpain, which needs to be associated with calpain-1 and calpain-2 to have a function). While calpain-1 and calpain-2 are present ubiquitously in all cells, the other members of the family have a more restricted distribution with some of them existing only in selected cell types[3]. Another major difference between the brain and the other organs/tissues is that neurons are the only cells that do not divide, unlike the majority of cells. An important clue to answer this question is provided by the calpain-1 knock-out mice. As we discussed, these mice are lacking calpain-1 globally and still they appear relatively normal, and one needs to use fine analysis to detect the problems they are exhibiting, which are mostly confined to brain functions. The exception is in fact the finding from Dr. Chishti, the "creator" of these mice, who found a defect in blood platelets, as they show enhanced spreading. These findings indicate that calpain-1 does not exert any unique functions in the majority of cells, which suggests that there is enough redundancy with other calpains for cells to function normally even in the absence of calpain-1. Nevertheless, calpain-1 has been implicated in other cell functions, such as phagocytosis[4], the ability of certain cells to engulf debris, microbes and viruses, and exocytosis, the ability of cells to secrete vesicles. All these functions are explained by the calpain-1-mediated cleavage of cytoskeletal proteins, as we discussed in various chapters.

What about calpain-2 then? Another clue for its function in cells other than neurons was provided by another one of our findings that in brain, calpain-2 is associated with the tyrosine phosphatase PTPN13 as we discussed in the previous Chapter. This protein was previously identified in other cells and given another name, FAP1 (Fas-associated protein 1)[5]. The function of this protein is to prevent cells for dying in a process called apoptosis, also known as programmed cell death, or cell suicide. This process is engaged under a multitude of different conditions both physiological and pathological. As we discussed, this protein is cleaved selectively by calpain-2 and loses its function. Consequently, when calpain-2 is activated, cells become much more susceptible to commit suicide. This finding confirms that calpain-2 is indeed a critical component of cell death both in the brain and throughout the organism. We also discussed the role of calpain-2 in the regulation of cell adhesion, in which calpain-2 stimulates the disassembly of focal adhesion points, again a deleterious effect on cell function. It appears that the major reason why calpain-2 has been maintained throughout evolution is that it is needed during the embryonic period, since deletion of calpain-2 in germ cells is lethal during embryogenesis[6]. I have searched the literature extensively and have yet to find evidence for a beneficial effect of calpain-2 after the embryonic period, strengthening the notion that indeed calpain-2 is a "bad enzyme."

This is rather good news, since an important issue for developing a novel drug is the question of side-effects, which represent a major reason why drugs fail in clinical trials, which are performed to identify potential side-effects. We were already encouraged by the results of a previous Phase I clinical trial in which a non-selective calpain inhibitor was tested for the treatment of Alzheimer's disease by Abbvie Pharmaceuticals. In the trial, the drug, Alicapistat, was given twice a day for 2 weeks to healthy subjects as well as patients with mild Alzheimer's disease. The results of the trial indicated that the drug did not produce significant side-effects as compared to the placebo[7]. However, the drug also did not produce any of the pharmacological effects the investigators were looking for and Abbvie did not pursue the development of Alicapistat for AD. As the study did not incorporate any marker for verifying the efficacy of the drug to inhibit calpain, it is difficult to conclude that the absence of side effects was due to the lack of potential side effects of calpain-2. This is why we are confident that our trial, which includes blood biomarkers reflecting brain calpain-2 activation, has a better chance to provide information regarding the efficacy of NA-184 to inhibit its target in the brain.

Another lesson learned is that great science is not the exclusivity of big labs and big universities. Throughout my career, I had a relatively small lab and even at the peak of my research activities the number of postdocs, Ph.D. students and undergraduate students working in my lab never exceeded a dozen people. This contrasts to the big labs who can have up to 50 people working. Quantification of science productivity is a difficult exercise and a number of metrics have been developed to attempt to rank scientists. For instance, one can use the number of publications a scientist has published, but this number does not necessarily reflect the impact of these publications. A parameter frequently used by scientists and administrators to evaluate the performance of faculty/researcher is the H-index, which represents the maximum number of publications (h) that have been cited at least h times by other scientists. Thus, an H-index of 100 means that the scientist has published at least 100 papers that have been cited at least 100 times. Now, it is clear that a large lab is likely to publish many more papers than a small lab, as more people are working in the lab. But more publications do not mean a higher H-index if these papers are not cited, which would indicate that these papers do not have a big impact in the field. The website Research.com provides a ranking of the best scientists in various fields based on what they call the D-index, which is a small modification of the H-index. The ranking is using data acquired on 06/12/2021 and is therefore somewhat outdated. I found myself ranked 819 in the World (433 in the US) with a D-index of 71, 17,550 citations for 188 publications. For comparison, the person ranked # 1, Dr. Trevor Robbins has a D-index of 234 with 174,455 citations for 843 publications. Dr. Eric Kandel, whom we mentioned at the beginning of the book is ranked # 6 with a D-index of 197 with 136,656 citations for 517 publications. Another web tool, Google Scholar also provides H-index for scientists. However, one has to be careful as these databases do not discriminate scientists with similar last names and first name initials. All of this is to emphasize that we currently do not have the tools to determine quantitatively what great science is. Mostly, time will be the judge, as great works survive while irrelevant work vanishes.

What would also be interesting to know is what is the cost of science, and how small groups and small universities contribute in comparison to large groups and large universities. Clearly, the bulk of the money spent on science goes to large labs and large universities. But does this mean that these large labs generate more relevant and impactful science than small ones, and what is the ratio cost/productivity? A recent publication analyzed what funding supports in terms of personnel, spending and publications[8]. It suggests that $100,000 results in 0.8 publication per year, i.e., the cost for 1 publication would be $125,000. I remember that when I started in Gary's lab, I was told that the cost for one publication was about $10,000. A rough estimate from my own numbers gave a value of $35,000 per publication. Again, these data suggest that it is possible to do great science and at a very reasonable cost in a small lab in a small university.

Finally, I need to reflect on the value of starting companies based on discoveries made in the lab. Both my Ph.D. advisor in France, JC Schwartz, and my postdoc advisor in the US, Gary Lynch, started companies. JC Schwartz started BioProjet (www.bioprojet.com) in 1982 after I already left the lab. Bioprojet was in part the result of work performed by my friend Bernard Malfroy who discovered the enzyme enkephalinase, which degrades the endogenous opioid peptides, which are the endogenous pain killers. This led to the development of an inhibitor for this enzyme, named Tiorfan used to treat diarrhea. Since then, Bioprojet has successfully launched Wakix, a blocker of a novel histamine receptor discovered by Jean-Charles lab, to treat narcolepsy, where patients fall asleep suddenly during daytime. Bioprojet has now many products and is a very successful, privately owned company.

As we discussed in the book, Gary Lynch started several companies. While Synaptics was a success, Gary Lynch did not really contribute to its development. Cortex Pharmaceuticals, which was started in 1986, is still functioning under the name of RespireRx Pharmaceuticals (www.respirerx.com), and has a molecule, CX-1739, in Phase I and Phase II clinical trials for a variety of indications, including spinal cord injury. On the other hand, the other two companies Gary started, Tensor Pharmaceuticals and Thorus, did not survive. Thus, there is still a chance that one of his companies will succeed in bringing a novel molecule for the treatment of a serious disorder.

Several of my friends and colleagues have also been involved in starting pharmaceutical companies. For example, Bernard started Eukarion, which became MindSetRx. Bernard is still pushing for the development of one of the EUK molecules for the treatment of rare diseases. Serge Bischoff started Rhenovia Pharma, which failed after 7 years. My colleague, Mark Bear, started Allos Pharma, previously Seaside Therapeutics, and the company is performing a Phase III clinical trial for fragile X syndrome, a neurodevelopmental disorder. One of Gary's graduate students who was in the lab when I was a postdoc there, later started a company, PhosphoSolutions, which manufactures and distributes antibodies for research applications, and has been very successful. In the field of neurosciences, Dr. Solomon Snyder, who won the Lasker Award in 1978, was involved in starting two pharmaceutical companies, Nova Pharmaceuticals and Guilford, who became very successful companies. Interestingly, Snyder's laboratory and Jean-Charles laboratory were fierce competitors in the search for the function of histamine in the brain when I was a graduate student, and I remember Snyder visiting Jean-Charles lab in the early 70s in Paris.

It is important to note that many large pharmaceutical companies have pulled back or cut down on the development of drugs for brain disorders, presumably due to the difficulties associated with such development. This is in large part due to the many failures in the field of Alzheimer's disease and stroke as well as other indications. These failures are clearly linked to the lack of understanding of the mechanisms involved in these diseases and the difficulties to find appropriate animal models of these diseases. As we discussed in the book, Alzheimer's disease has been cured many times in mouse models but these findings have not translated into success in the human disease. Only recent developments have produced potential therapeutic approaches that appear to slow down the progression of the disease. These approaches consist in administering antibodies against ß-amyloid, which clear the amyloid plaques from the brain[9]. Thus, it is up to small biotech companies to perform the bulk of the initial drug development for neurological and neuropsychiatric disorders. By and large these biotech companies are the result of academic research and the conviction by academic neuroscientists that their discoveries can indeed have a profound impact on the health of millions of people. This has indeed been my drive all throughout the last 45 years, and while the story is not finished, I am still hopeful that these 45 years of research will result in a drug that will prevent the devastating consequences of concussions. As we also discussed, it could also benefit other disorders associated with neurodegeneration. The next 5 years will indeed tell us if this prediction is right.

ACKNOWLEDGMENTS

I need to thank so many people who, one way or another, have been helping me in my long journey towards finding a cure for TBI and other neurodegenerative diseases. It all started with Bernard Roques at Ecole Polytechnique, who planted the seeds of research in my mind, and his advice to study biochemistry paid off. The 7 years spent in the laboratory of Jean-Charles Schwartz transformed me from an unsophisticated graduate student into an ambitious scientist ready to make big discoveries. Serge Bischoff first taught me how to run biological experiments. Later, he taught me how to transform basic findings into clinical applications. Throughout the years he has been a great friend. Jean-Pierre Changeux was one of the members of my dissertation committee and has been a role model ever since I met him. Gary Lynch has been a mentor, a collaborator and a friend for more than 40 years now, and I would not be where I am now without him. He taught me not to be afraid of thinking big and to explore new frontiers (in addition to understanding the subtleties of baseball). Bernard Malfroy has been a constant friend, collaborator, and partner in various projects since 1988, and we have shared the ups and downs of both the research process and of its translation to clinical applications. Richard/Dick Thompson was instrumental to bring me to USC from UC Irvine, a move that proved to be invaluable. I could never thank my wife,

Xiaoning Bi, enough. Ever since she entered my life, she has been my sunshine, my soulmate and my best collaborator, and she has helped me benefit from all the failures I experienced. Michael Palfreyman has been a constant source of support and advice. His vast experience in pharma and biotech and his large network of talented people have been critical to create NeurAegis and to make it thrive and successful.

Athar Chishti provided us the calpain-1 knock-out mice, which have been an incredible tool to help us understand what calpain-1 and calpain-2 are doing in the brain. Yubin Wang was an outstanding scientist who made the majority of the breakthrough discoveries from the lab over the last 10 years. I also need to thank the three research assistant professors who worked with me at USC, Drs. Georges Tocco, Juan Carlos Marvizon and Hussam Jourdi, and made significant contributions to the work I described in the book. Between UCI, USC and WesternU, I have trained and worked with 20 postdoctoral scholars, without whom the work could not have been done. Likewise, the 39 graduate students who worked in my various labs made enormous contributions to our understanding of the roles of calpains in the brain. Throughout the years, an army of undergraduate students provided the hard and repetitive work representing the 99% perspiration of the research process, and I hope that their lab experience made a difference in their careers.

I want to thank all the people who agreed to work with us at NeurAegis and have spent hours and hours helping us make our dream of bringing a selective calpain-2 inhibitors to the clinic come true. Philippe Bey, Norton Peet, Shujaath Mehdi, Joe Blanchard, Kathy Fosnaugh and Greg Coulter. Stella Sung, my co-author, has been an outstanding CEO, and her faith in our project is unshakable.

Greg DiRienzo, one of NeurAegis co-founders, has been a constant source of mental support and was instrumental in introducing us to Alan Morell.

I also need to thank all the funding agencies and other private sources of funding who provided the necessary means to perform the work. These include the NIH, the NSF, the Alzheimer's Association and the Department of Defense.

Finally, I need to give special thanks to all the people who shared my life and my dreams over the years. Of these, my two children, Neema and Tara Baudry, as well as Xiaoning's daughter, Angela Ji, have a unique place in my heart and remind us that nothing important can be done without unconditional love.

ADDITIONAL READINGS

The Neuroscience of Traumatic Brain Injury
1st Edition - July 29, 2022
Editors: Rajkumar Rajendram, Victor Preedy, Colin Martin
Publisher: Elsevier

Shaken Brain: The Science, Care, and Treatment of Concussion
Hardcover – Illustrated, February 11, 2020
by Elizabeth Sandel MD (Author)
Publisher: Harvard University Press

Understanding Traumatic Brain Injury: A Guide for Survivors and Families
Paperback – September 27, 2021
by Richard H. Adler (Author)
Publisher: World Association Publishers

The Traumatized Brain: A Family Guide to Understanding Mood, Memory, and Behavior after Brain Injury (A Johns Hopkins Press Health Book) Illustrated Edition
by Vani Rao (Author), Sandeep Vaishnavi (Author), Peter V. Rabins (Foreword)
Publisher: Johns Hopkins Press

Mild Traumatic Brain Injury and Postconcussion Syndrome: The New Evidence Base for Diagnosis and Treatment
by **Michael A. McCrea**
2007 Oxford University

ABOUT THE AUTHORS; DR. MICHEL BAUDRY AND DR. STELLA SUNG

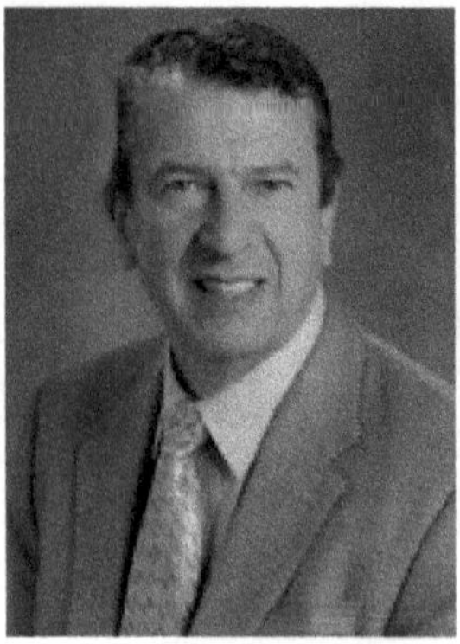

Dr. Michel Baudry is currently Professor of Biomedical Sciences in the Graduate College of Biomedical Sciences at Western University of Health Sciences in Pomona, CA. His previous position was Professor of Biological Sciences, Neurology and Biomedical Engineering at USC, Los Angeles, CA. After graduating from the prestigious Ecole Polytechnique in Paris (France) in 1971, Baudry obtained a Ph.D. in Biochemistry at the University of Paris VII in 1977. In 1978 he moved to the US for a postdoctoral period with Prof. Gary Lynch at UC Irvine. He remained at UCI as an Assistant and then an Associate Professor until 1989, before moving to USC in 1989.

Dr. Baudry is a world-known neuroscientist and has published over 400 manuscripts in peer-reviewed journals. He is one of the 100 most cited neuroscientists, according to the ISI database. In collaboration with Prof. Lynch, Baudry developed a biochemical theory for Learning and Memory that is still one of the most widely accepted theories in the field. Baudry's research is directed at understanding the molecular mechanisms of learning and memory as well as those involved in neurodegenerative processes underlying numerous human brain diseases.

Dr. Baudry has also been involved in several start-up companies. In 1986 he was one of the co-founders of Synaptics, Inc, the Human Interface company. In 1991, he co-founded Eukarion, Inc, and more recently participated in the transformation of Eukarion into MindSet, Rx. In 2007, he also co-founded Rhenovia Pharma, a drug discovery & development company located in Mulhouse, France. Finally, in February 2016, in collaboration with several faculty members at WesternU and entrepreneurs, he started NeurAegis, Inc, a neuroscience company directed at developing neuroprotective drugs for the treatment of a variety of neurodegenerative diseases.

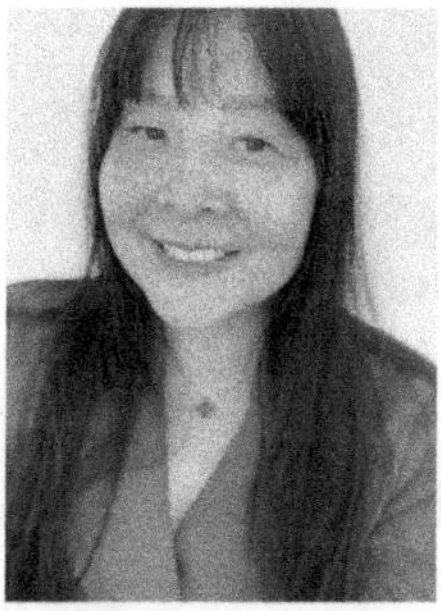

Dr. Stella Sung is a life science/biotech executive with 25 years of experience in both operating and venture capital roles. She is the CEO of NeurAegis, Inc. as well as a member of its Board of Directors. Dr. Sung has been a "C-level" executive (CEO/CBO) at multiple life science companies, including AEGEA Biotechnologies, Decoy Biosystems, ImmunoActiva, Tauriga Sciences, Avita Medical, PliCare Therapeutics and Cylene Pharmaceuticals. Dr. Sung has negotiated numerous transactions, agreements, and partnerships, and she has structured and led financings. She also has built companies as a venture investor. Dr. Sung has a successful track record as a General Partner or Managing Director at several venture firms, including Oxford Bioscience Partners, Coastview Capital and Pearl St. Venture Fund, where her experience also includes ten Board of Directors positions, including five as Chairperson of the Board. Dr. Sung received her Ph.D. in chemistry from Harvard University, where she was a National Science Foundation Predoctoral Fellow, and her B.S. in chemistry with a minor in English from Ohio State University, *Phi Beta Kappa*.

GLOSSARY SECTION

ADME: Absorption, Distribution, Metabolism, Excretion: terms used for characterizing how molecules are processed following administration.

C2I: Calpain-2 Inhibitor: initial inhibitor resulting from the work at Cortex Pharmaceuticals.

Calpain: a family of calcium-dependent proteases, which cleave many proteins, thereby modifying their functions.

CCI: Controlled Cortical Impact: animal model of open skull brain injury

CMC: Chemistry, Manufacturing and Control: covers the various procedures used to assess the physical and chemical characteristics of drug products.

CTE: Chronic Traumatic Encephalopathy

CV: Coefficient of Variation: statistical measure of the dispersion of data points around their means

IND: Investigational New Drug: IND application to the FDA is required before initiating clinical trials.

i.p.: intraperitoneal: mode of drug delivery in experimental animals.

i.v.: intravenous: use for drug delivery in animals and humans.

KO: Knock-Out: mouse strain genetically modified to lack a specific gene.

Log (P): Partition coefficient for n-octanol/water: represents the solubility of molecules in tissues.

MW: Molecular Weight: the weight of 1 mole of a molecule

NFL: National Football League

PK/PD: Pharmacokinetic/Pharmacodynamic: represent the rate of elimination of a molecule/the rate of disappearance of the effect of a molecule.

SBDP: Spectrin BreakDown Product: used as a marker of calpain activation.

SNTF: Spectrin N-Terminal Fragment: used as a blood biomarker of brain calpain activation.

TBI: Traumatic Brain Injury: also called concussion, which can be mild, moderate or severe

WT: Wild-type: normal mouse strain.

CAST OF CHARACTERS

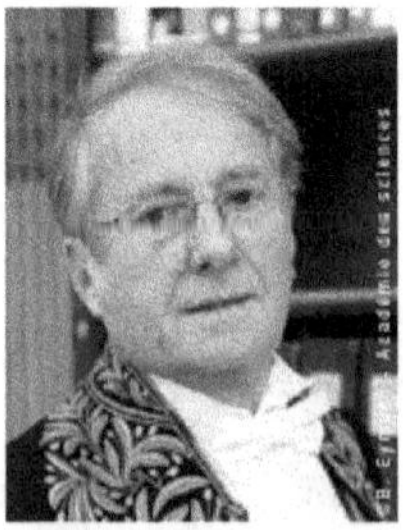

Jean-Charles Schwartz: (born 1936) French pharmacist and neurobiologist. Director of INSERM U-109. Co-Founder of Bioprojet. Member of the French National Academy of Sciences.

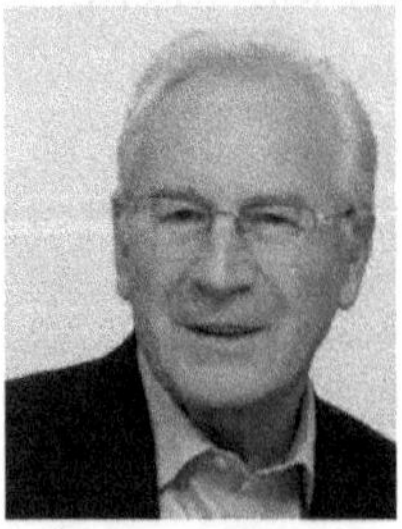

Bernard Roques: (born 1935) French pharmacist, pharmacologist, Chair of Pharmaco-chemistry at the University of Pharmacy, Paris, France. Member of the National French Academy of Sciences. Co-founder Pharmaleads.

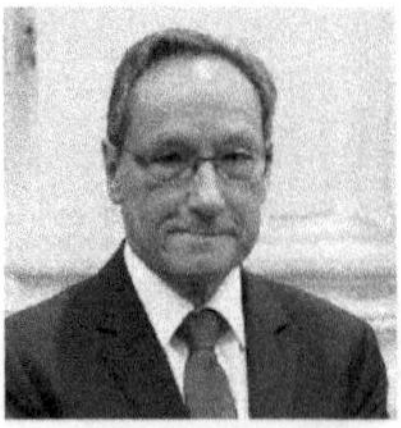

Serge Bischoff: (born 1948) French neurobiologist. Co-founder of Rhenovia Pharma. Laureate of the Grand Prix 2015 Emilia Valori of the French Academy of Sciences

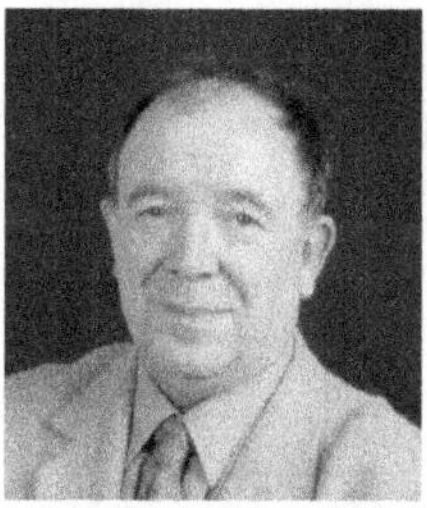

Jean-Pierre Changeux: (born 1936) French neurobiologist, Professor, College de France, Member of the French National Academy of Sciences and of the American National Academy of Sciences. Author of many books, including "The neuronal man."

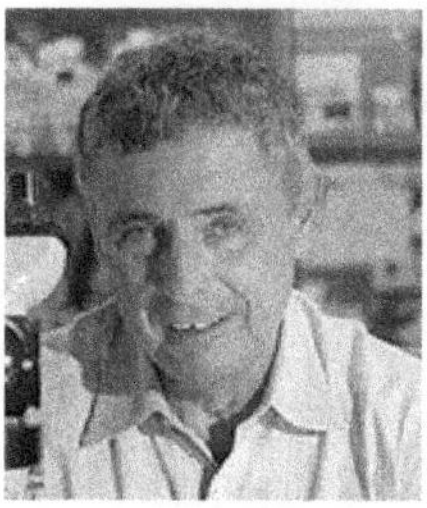

Gary Lynch: (born 1943) American neurobiologist. Professor of Psychiatry and Human Behavior, UC Irvine. Co-founder of Synaptics, Cortex Pharmaceuticals, Tensor and Thuris. Author of: "Big brain: the origin and evolution of human intelligence."

Takashi Murachi

Takashi Murachi: (1926-1990) Professor and Chairman of the Department of Clinical Science and Laboratory Medicine, Kyoto University.

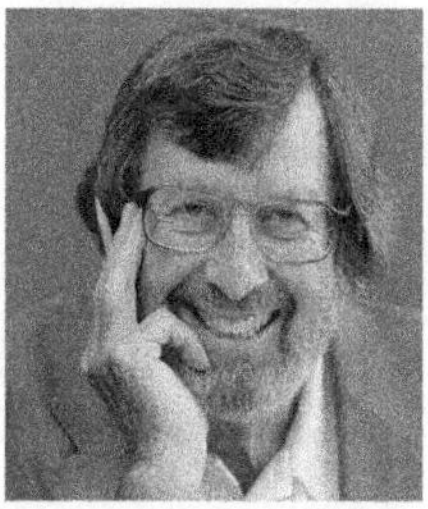

Richard Thompson: (1930-2014) American neuroscientist. Director of the Center for Neural, Information and Behavioral Sciences, USC. Member of the American National Academy of Sciences.

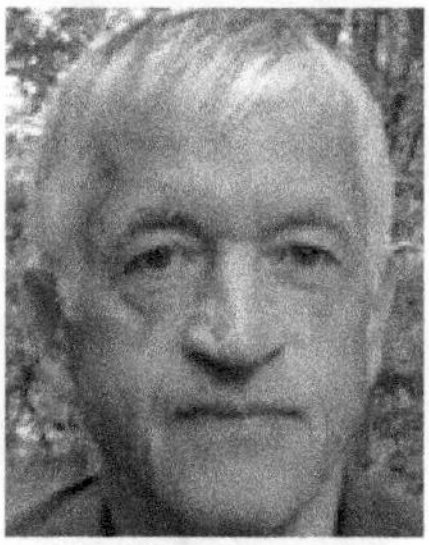

Bernard Malfroy-Camine: (born 1953) French neurobiologist. Co-founder of Eukarion, MindSet and NeurAegis. Author of: "The marathon man."

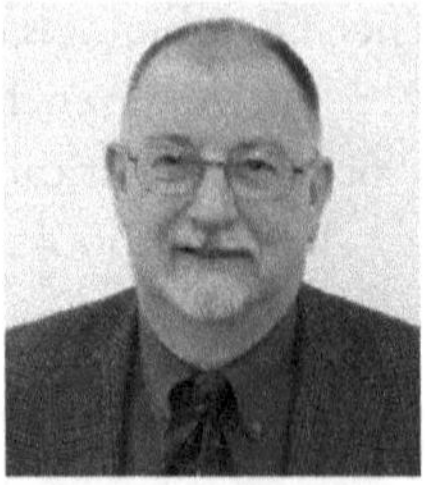

Michael Palfreyman: (born 1945) Leader in biotechnology and pharmaceutical industries. Co-founded numerous biotech companies. Chief R&D Officer, Cybin.

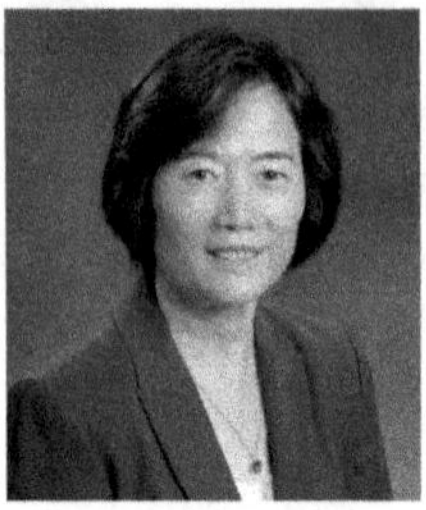

Xiaoning Bi: (born 1960) American neurobiologist. Professor of Basic Medical Sciences, Western University of Health Sciences, Pomona. Co-founder NeurAegis.

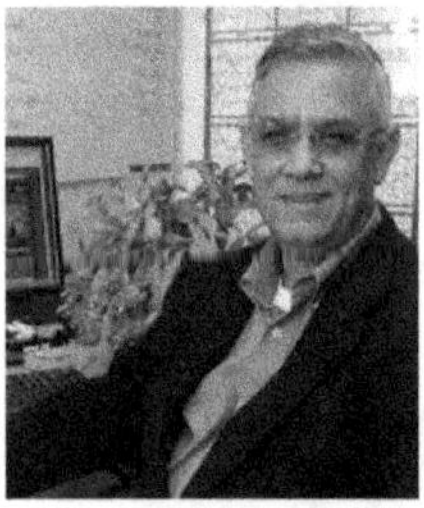

Athar Chishti: (born 1957) American biochemist, Professor of Molecular and Chemical Biology, Tufts University, Boston. Founder of Calpgen Therapeutics. Made the calpain-1 knock out mice.

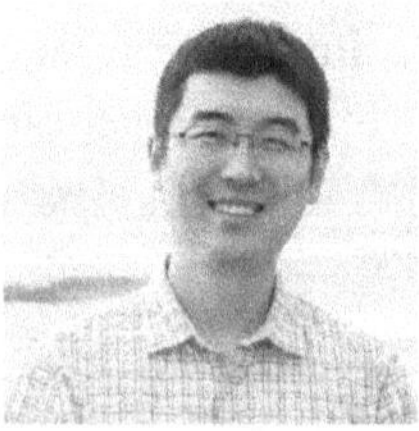

Yubin Wang: (born 1984) Neurobiologist. Co-founder NeurAegis. Currently work at Mabwell Therapeutics.

NOTES AND REFERENCES

NOTES AND REFERENCES FOR CHAPTER 1

1. Ecole Polytechnique: the school was founded in 1794 by the French mathematician, Gaspard Monge and became militarized under Napoleon in 1804. The original school was located in Paris but moved to the Paris suburb of Saclay/Palaiseau in 1976.
2. Merrifield peptide synthesis: Bruce Merrifield developed the solid-phase peptide synthesis which involves attaching the C-terminus of the peptide chain to a polymeric solid. Amino acids are added to the N-terminus.
3. Baudry, M., Martres, M.P. and Schwartz, J.C. H1- and H2-receptors in the histamine-induced accumulation of cyclic AMP in guinea-pig cortical slices. *Nature* **253:** 362-363, 1975.
4. "Apprentices of Wonder: Inside the Neural Network Revolution." William F. Allman. Bantam. 1989.
5. Synaptics, Inc. The company was founded in 1986 and was initially called the Minos Corporation. It was renamed Synaptics in 1987 and is located in San Jose, CA.
6. Touchpad. This is the device used on many laptops to move the cursor on the screen.

7. https://www.defensemedianetwork.com/stories/taking-neurotechnology-new-territory/
8. AI. Artificial Intelligence started as the simulation of human intelligence with computers. Currently, it is a field, which combines computer science and database analysis to solve a variety of complex problems.
9. Neurotechnologies. The term refers to all technologies that help understand the brain and nervous system activity or affect brain and nervous system functions.
10. https://braininitiative.nih.gov
11. Ampakines. Ampakines are positive allosteric modulators of the AMPA receptors, a subtype of the glutamate receptors. They enhance the responses of the receptors when glutamate binds to the receptors.
12. Cephalon, Inc. Cephalon initial research focus was on developing a treatment for amyotrophic lateral sclerosis (ALS, aka Lou Gehrig's disease). It then marketed Provigil for the treatment of sleep disorders.
13. **Siman et al. "Evidence That the Blood Biomarker SNTF Predicts Brain Imaging Changes and Persistent Cognitive Dysfunction in Mild TBI Patients."** ***Front Neurol.*** **4: 190. 2013.**
14. Alkermes. Alkermes was founded in 1987 and focuses on central nervous system diseases. In 2011, it merged with a division of Elan Corporation.
15. SOD/catalase. Superoxide dismutase and catalase are the main enzymes that detoxify oxygen free radicals in leaving organisms. While SOD produces H_2O_2 from the oxygen free radical, catalase transforms H_2O_2 into water and oxygen.
16. Gilbert Chauvet: "La vie dans la matière: le role de l'espace en biologie." Flamarion. 1998.
17. Serge Bischoff: Laureat du prix Emilia Valori for science applications, 2015.
18. Calpains. A 15-member family of calcium-dependent proteases. Calpain-1 and calpain-2 were the first members of the family identified and are called the classical calpains. They are found ubiquitously in cells and tissues from almost all living organisms.

19. Limitless. This 2011 movie stars Bradley Cooper and Robert de Niro and is based on the discovery of a pill that enhances brain abilities.
20. DFMO. Difluoromethylornithine is an inhibitor of ornithine decarboxylase and is an anti-parasitic agent and inhibitor of mammalian cell growth.
21. NIH Blueprint. The NIH Blueprint for neuroscience research is designed to accelerate research and development of new therapies for brain disorders.

NOTES AND REFERENCES FOR CHAPTER 2

1. https://ncschweitzerfellowship.org/an-invisible-injury-visibly-impacting-athletes/
2. "From scientist to salesman." Will Hobson. *Washington Post*, Jan, 22, 2020.
3. https://www.globalpointofcare.abbott/en/product-details/apoc/istat-tbi-plasma.html
4. NNZ-2566. "Mechanism of action for NNZ-2566 anti-inflammatory effects following PBBI involves upregulation of immunomodulator ATF3." Cartagena et al., *Neuromolecular Medicine*, 15: 504-514. 2013.
5. Excitotoxicity. A series of deleterious events initiated by an excessive release of the excitatory neurotransmitter glutamate.
6. **"The use of repetitive transcranial magnetic stimulation (rTMS) following traumatic brain injury (TBI): A scoping review." Pink et al., *Neuropsychology Rehabilitation*, 31: 479-505, 2021.**
7. **"Hyperbaric oxygen therapy for traumatic brain injury: bench-to-bedside.." Hu et al., *Medical Gas Research*. 6: 102-110, 2016.**
8. "Stem cell therapy for sequestration of traumatic brain injury-induced inflammation." Borlogan and Rosi. *International Journal of Molecular Sciences*. 23(18):10286, 2022.

9. **"Cell Therapy for Chronic TBI: Interim Analysis of the Randomized Controlled STEMTRA Trial." Kawabori et al.,** *Neurology* **4: 1202-1214, 2021.**
10. **"Editorial: Brain Hypoxia and Ischemia: New Insights Into Neurodegeneration and Neuroprotection." Nalivaeva and Rybnikova.** *Frontiers in Neurosciences*, **13:770, 2019.**
11. CT scan. Computerized tomography (CT) scan uses a series of X-ray images to create a 3D-model of the area examined, such as the brain. It is widely used to examine patients who have suffered TBI to diagnose the extent of the injury.
12. Hardingham, GE. "Coupling of the NMDA receptor to neuro-protective and neurodestructive events." *Biochem Soc Trans*. 37: 1147-1160. 2009.
13. Wang et al. "Protection against TBI-induced neuronal death with post-treatment with a selective calpain-2 inhibitor in mice." *J. Neurotrauma*, **34:** 1-13, 2018.
14. Inflammation. Body response to protect against infection or heal from an insult or injury. Mediated by white blood cells and the chemicals they release.
15. Blood cells involved in immune responses consist of macro-phages, neutrophils, monocytes and natural killer cells. These cells circulate throughout the body and react rapidly after an injury.
16. "How neuroinflammation contributes to neurodegeneration." Ransoff RM. *Science*, 353: 777-783. 2016.
17. "A clinical trial of progesterone for severe traumatic brain injury." Skolnick et al., *The New England Journal of Medicine*, 371: 2467-2476, 2014.
18. https://www.clinicaltrialsarena.com/news/vasopharm-ronopterin-fails-trial/
19. Wang et al. "Calpain-2 as a therapeutic target for acute neuronal injury." *Expert Opinion in Therapeutic Target,* 22: 19-29, 2018.
20. Wang et al. "P13BP, a calpain-2-mediated breakdown product of PTPN13, is a novel blood biomarker for traumatic brain injury." *Journal of Neurotrauma,* 2021. DOI: 10.1089/neu.2021.0229.

NOTES AND REFERENCES FOR CHAPTER 3

1. Bliss TV and Lomo T. "Long-lasting potentiation of synaptic transmission in the dentate area of the anaesthetized rabbit following stimulation of the perforant path." *J Physiol.* 232: 331-356. 1973.
2. Lynch G et al. "Long-term potentiation is accompanied by a reduction in dendritic responsiveness to glutamic acid." *Nature.* 263: 151-153. 1976.
3. Baudry et al. "Decreased responsiveness to low doses of apomorphine and the possible involvement of hyposensitivity of dopamine autoreceptors." *Neuroscience Letters* 4: 203-207, 1977.
4. Lynch et al. "Intracellular injections of EGTA block induction of hippocampal long-term potentiation." *Nature* 305: 719-721. 1983.
5. Baudry M and Lynch G. "Regulation of glutamate receptors by cations." *Nature.* 282: 748-750. 1979.
6. Cysteine or thiol proteases have a cysteine amino acid in their catalytic site, which means they are using the thiol, SH, group to attack the peptide bond in the target protein.
7. Baudry et al. "Micromolar levels of calcium stimulate proteolytic activity and glutamate receptor binding in rat brain synaptic membranes." *Science* **212:** 937-938, 1981.
8. Siman, R., Baudry, M. and Lynch, G. "Brain fodrin: Substrate for calpain I, an endogenous calcium-activated protease." *Proc. Natl. Acad. Sci.* (USA) **81:** 3572-3576, 1984.
9. https://en.wikipedia.org/wiki/Spectrin.
10. Lynch, G. and Baudry, M. "The biochemistry of memory: A new and specific hypothesis." *Science.* **224:** 1057-1063, 1984.
11. Johnson G. "In the palaces of memory: How we build the Worlds inside our heads." Random House, New York. 1991.
12. A J-1 visa provide exchange opportunities in research or cultural and educational programs. Such a visa is for a duration of up to 3 years. A two-year home residency requirement is imposed if the home country funds the research. A H-1 visa is used for

temporary employment visitors and for those who intend to apply for permanent residency.

13. Mamounas et al. "Classical conditioning of the rabbit eyelid response increases glutamate receptor binding in hippocampal synaptic membranes." *Proc. Natl. Acad. Sci.* (USA) **81:** 2548-2552, 1984.
14. De Luca SN, Sominsky L and Spencer SJ. Delayed spatial win-shift on radial arm maze. *Bio-protocol* 6 (23) e2053. DOI: 10.21769/BioProtoc.2053.
15. Staubli, U., Baudry, M. and Lynch, G. "Leupeptin, a thiol-protease inhibitor causes a selective impairment of maze performance in rats." *Behav. Neural Biol.* **40:** 58-69, 1984.
16. Staubli, U., Baudry, M. and Lynch, G. "Olfactory discrimination learning is blocked by leupeptin, a thiol protease inhibitor." *Brain Res.* **337:** 333-336, 1985.
17. Morris et al. "Spatial learning in the rat: Impairments induced by the thiol-proteinase inhibitor, leupeptin, and an analysis of [^{3}H]-glutamate receptor binding in relation to learning." *Behav. Neural Biol.* **5:** 333-345, 1987.
18. Long-term depression. This phenomenon was reported in 1992 by Serena Dudek and Mark Bear "Homosynaptic long-term depression in area CA1 of hippocampus and effects of N-methyl-D-aspartate receptor blockade." *Proc. Nat. Acad. Sci.* 89: 4363-4367. Since then, many studies have been devoted to understand the function of this phenomenon in learning and memory, but have not provided a clear answer.

NOTES AND REFERENCES FOR CHAPTER 4

1. https://en.wikipedia.org/wiki/Cloning#:~:text=Cloning%20is%20the%20process%20of,cells%20and%20of%20DNA%20fragments.
2. Bochet, P. and Rossier, J. Molecular biology of excitatory amino acid receptors: subtypes and subunits. *EXS*. 1993;63:224-33. doi: 10.1007/978-3-0348-7265-2_10.

3. Baudry, M., Su, W. and Bi, X. "The Calpain Proteolytic System." In Bradshaw Ralph A., Hart Gerald W. and Stahl Philip D. (eds.) *Encyclopedia of Cell Biology, Second Edition, vol. 1*, 2023, pp. 852–864. Oxford: Elsevier.
4. Isoforms. A **protein isoform**, or "**protein variant**", is a member of a set of highly similar proteins that originate from a single gene or gene family.
5. Ionotropic receptors. Ionotropic receptors are ligand-gated ion channels made up of three, four, or five protein subunits that together form an ion-conducting pore in the center of the receptor.
6. https://www.orpha.net/consor/cgi-bin/OC_Exp.php?lng=EN&Expert=267#:~:text=A%20subtype%20of%20autosomal%20recessive,compartment%20of%20the%20limbs%20are
7. Nowak, L., Bregetovki, P., Ascher, P., Herbet, A. and Prochiantz, A. Magnesium gates glutamate-activated channels in mouse central neurones. *Nature*, 307: 462-465, 1984.
8. Morris, R.G.M., Anderson, E., Lynch, G.S. and Baudry, M. "Selective impairment of learning and blockade of long-term potentiation by N-methyl-D-aspartate receptor antagonist, AP-5." *Nature* **319:** 774-776, 1986.
9. Morris, R.G.M. et al. "Spatial learning in the rat: Impairments induced by the thiol-proteinase inhibitor, leupeptin, and an analysis of [^{3}H]-glutamate receptor binding in relation to learning." *Behav. Neural Biol.* **5:** 333-345, 1987.
10. Kessler, M., Petersen, G., Vu, M.H., Baudry, M. and Lynch, G. PHE-GLU stimulated, chloride-dependent glutamate "binding" represents glutamate sequestration mediated by an exchange system. *J. Neurochem.* **48:** 1191-1200, 1987.
11. Lisman, J. A mechanism for the Hebb and anti-Hebb processes underlying learning and memory. *Proc. Nat Acad Sci USA.* 86: 9574-9578. 1989.
12. Lynch, G. and Baudry, M. Brain spectrin, calpain and long-term changes in synaptic efficacy. *Brain Res. Bull.* **18:** 809-815, 1987.

13. Lee, K. et al. Brief bursts of high frequency stimulation produce two types of structural change in rat hippocampus. *J. Neurophysiol.* 44: 247-258, 1980.

NOTES AND REFERENCES FOR CHAPTER 5

1. Lynch G. and Baudry, M. The origins and manifestation of neuronal plasticity in the hippocampus. In The Clinical Neurosciences, vol. 5 Neurobiology. (Series editor Roger N Rosenberg. Associate Editor William D. Willis. 1983. Churchill Livingstone, New York. pg 171-202.
2. Ivy G. et al. "Lesions of entorhinal cortex produce a calpain-mediated degradation of brain spectrin in dentate gyrus. II. Anatomical studies." *Brain Res.* **459:** 233-240, 1988.
3. Bi, X., Chang, V., Tocco, G. and Baudry, M. Regional distribution and time-course of calpain activation following kainate-induced seizure activity in adult rat brain. *Brain Res.* **726:** 98-108, 1996.
4. Lynch, G. and Baudry, M. Structure-function relationships in the organization of memory." In: "Perspectives in Memory Research." (M. Gazzaniga, ed.), MIT Press, Cambridge, MA, 1988, pp. 23-91.
5. Cooper, L.N. and Scofield, C.L. "Mean-field theory of a neural network." *Proc. Nat. Acad. Sci. USA.* 85: 1973-1977, 1973.
6. Granger, R.et al. "Non-hebbian properties of long-term potentiation enable high-capacity encoding of temporal sequences."" *Proc. Nat. Acad. Sci. USA.* 91: 10104-10108, 1994.
7. Lynch G. and Granger R. "Big brain: the origins and future of human intelligence." St Martin's Griffin. New York. 2008.
8. Baudry, M. and Lynch, G. Properties and substrates of mammalian memory systems. In: "Psychopharmacology, Third Generation of Progress." (H.Y. Meltzer, ed), New York, Raven Press, 1987, 449-462.
9. Baudry, M., DuBrin, R., Beasley, L., Leon, M. and Lynch, G. Low levels of calpain in Chiroptera brain: Implications for mechanisms of aging. *Neurobiol. Aging* **9:** 255-258, 1986.

10. Professors-in-Residence are academically qualified research or other creative personnel who engage in teaching, research, and University service to the same extent as those holding the corresponding titles in the professorial series in the same department.
11. Petanque. Sports into the category of boules sports. https://en.wikipedia.org/wiki/P%C3%A9tanque
12. Taubes G. "Nobel dreams: Power, deceit and the ultimate experiment." Random House, 1987.

NOTES AND REFERENCES FOR CHAPTER 6

1. Malfroy-Camine B. Marathoning through life. Amazon, 2018.
2. Ataxia Telangiectasia (AT)—also known as Louis-Bar syndrome, cerebello-oculocutaneous telangiectasia, or immunodeficiency with ataxia telangiectasia—is a rare inherited childhood neurological disorder that affects the part of the brain that controls motor movement (intended movement of muscles) and speech.
3. Massicotte, G., Vanderklish, P., Lynch, G., and Baudry, M. Modulation of AMPA/quisqualate receptors by phospholipase A2: A necessary step in long-term potentiation? *Proc. Nat. Acad. Sci.* (USA) **88:** 1893-1897, 1991.
4. Beyer, W.F. and Fridovich, I. Characterization of a superoxide dismutase mimic prepared from desferrioxamine and MnO_2. *Arch. Biochem. Biophys.* 271: 149-156, 1989.
5. Baudry, M., Etienne, S., Bruce, A., Palucki, M., Jacobsen, E. and Malfroy, B. Salen-manganese complexes are superoxide dismutase-mimics. *Biochem. Biophys. Res. Comm.* **192:** 964-968,1993.
6. Melov, S. et al. Extension of lifespan with superoxide dismutase/catalase mimetics. Science. 289: 1567-1569. 2000.
7. Bi, X., Tocco, G. and Baudry, M. Calpain-mediated regulation of AMPA receptors in adult rat brain. *NeuroReport*. **6:** 61-64, 1994.
8. Bi, X., Chen, J., Dang, S., Wang, Z. and Baudry, M. Calpain-mediated regulation of NMDA receptor structure and function. *Brain Res.* **790:** 245-253, 1998.

9. Lu, X., Rong, Y. and Baudry, M. Calpain-mediated degradation of PSD-95 in developing and adult rat brain. *Neurosci. Lett.* **286:** 149-153, 2000.
10. Kandel, E.R. and Tauc, L. Mechanism of prolonged heterosynaptic facilitation. *Nature* 202: 145-147, 1964.
11. Baudry, M. and Lynch, G. Remembrance of arguments past: how well is the glutamate receptor hypothesis of LTP holding up after 20 years. *Neurobiol. Learning & Memory* **76:** 284-297, 2001.

NOTES AND REFERENCES FOR CHAPTER 7

1. McDermot, T. 101 Theory Drive: A Neuroscientist Quest for MEMORY. Pantheon Book, New York. 2010.
2. Shimono, K., Baudry, M., Ho, L., Taketani, M. and Lynch, G. Long term recording of LTP in cultured hippocampal slices. *Neural Plasticity.* 9: 249-254, 2002.
3. eCube™ is a novel EEG based discovery platform that probes the effects of compounds of different drug classes on electrical brain activity. eCube™ provides a uniform testing platform to record actigraphy and quantitative EEG (Q-EEG) and local field potentials (LFPs) from four brain regions of unanesthetized mice before and after drug administration. Similar to the SmartCube® process, raw data and the derived features from the brain signals and biometrics are used to train a machine learning classifier, which can be used to identify novel compounds with the desired EEG activity. Likewise, eCube™ can be used to phenotype disease models including autism spectral disorders, rare genetic epilepsies, HD, AD, and more. As EEG yields objective pharmaco-dynamic signatures specific to pharmacological action it can be used to evaluate translational biomarkers in CNS disorders and rapidly screen compounds for potential activity at specific pharmacological targets to provide valuable information for guiding the early stages of drug development.
4. Jourdi, H., Yanagihara, T., Martinez, U., Bi, X., Lynch, G. and Baudry, M. Effects of positive AMPA receptor modulators on

calpain-mediated spectrin degradation in cultured hippocampal slices. *Neurochem. Internat.* 46: 31-40, 2005.

5. Lauterborn, J.C. et al. Positive modulation of AMPA receptors increases neurotrophin expression by hippocampal and cortical neurons. *J. Neurosci.* 20: 8-21, 2000.
6. Thoenen, H. Neurotrophins and neuronal plasticity. *Science* 270: 593-598, 1005.
7. Crocker SJ et al. Inhibition of calpains prevents neuronal and behavioral deficits in an MPTP mouse model of Parkinson's disease. *J. Neurosci.* 23: 4081-4091, 2003.

NOTES AND REFERENCES FOR CHAPTER 8

1. Gene knock-out: A knockout, as related to genomics, refers to the use of genetic engineering to inactivate or remove one or more specific genes from an organism. Scientists create knockout organisms to study the impact of removing a gene from an organism, which often allows them to then learn something about that gene's function.

2. Azam, et al. Disruption of the mouse mu-calpain gene reveals an essential role in platelet function. *Mol. Cell Biol.* 21: 2213-2220, 2001.
3. Grammer, M., Kuchay, S., Chishti, A. and Baudry, M. Lack of phenotype for LTP and fear conditioning learning in calpain I knock-out mice. *Neurobiol. Learning and Memory*. **84:** 222-227, 2005.
4. Sterniczuk, R. et al. Characterization of the 3xTg-AD mouse model of Alzheimer's disease: Part 1. Circadian changes. *Brain Res.* 1348: 139-148, 2010.
5. Clausen, A., Xu, X., Bi, X. and Baudry, M. Effects of the superoxide dismutase/catalase mimetic EUK-207 in a mouse model of Alzheimer's disease: Protection against and interruption of progression of amyloid and tau pathology and cognitive decline. *J. Alz. Dis.* **30:** 183-208, 2012.
6. Clausen, A., Doctrow, S. and Baudry, M. Prevention of cognitive deficits and brain oxidative stress with superoxide dismutase/

catalase mimetics in aged mice. *Neurobiol. Aging*, **31:** 425-433, 2010.

7. Ambert, N., Greget, R., Haeberle, O., Bischoff, S., Berger, T.W., Bouteiller, J.M. and Baudry, M. Computational studies of NMDA receptors: differential effect of neuronal activity on potency of competitive and non-competitive antagonists. *Open Access BioInformatics*, **2010:2**: 113-125. 2010.
8. Bouteiller, J.M., Allam, S.L., Greget, R., Ambert, N. Hu, E.Y., Bischoff, S., Baudry, M. and Berger, T.W. Paired-pulse stimulation at glutamatergic synapses – pre- and post-synaptic components. *Conf Proc IEEE Eng Med Biol Soc*, 2010: 787-790, 2010.

NOTES AND REFERENCES FOR CHAPTER 9

1. Xu, W., Wong, T.P., Chery, N., Gaertner, T., Wang, Y.T. and Baudry, M. Calpain-mediated truncation of mGluR1a: a key step in excitotoxicity. *Neuron*, **53:** 399-412, 2007.
2. Xu, W., Zhou, M. and Baudry, M. Neuroprotection by cell permeable TAT-mGluR1 peptide in ischemia: synergy between carrier and cargo sequences. *NeuroScientist,* **14:** 409-414, 2008.
3. Glading, A. et al. Epidermal growth factor activates m-calpain (calpain II), at least in part, by extracellular signal-regulated kinase-mediated phosphorylation. *Mol. Cell Biol.* 24: 2499-2512, 2004.
4. Zadran, S., Jourdi, H., Rostamiani, K., Qin, Q., Bi, X. and Baudry, M. BDNF- and EGF-mediated neuronal calpain activation through MAPK-dependent phosphorylation. *J. Neurosci.* **30:** 1086-1095, 2010.
5. Zadran, S., Bi, X. and Baudry, M. Regulation of calpain-2 in neurons: Implications for synaptic plasticity. *Mol. Neurobiol.* 42:143-150, 2010.

NOTES AND REFERENCES FOR CHAPTER 10

1. Oliver, M., Baudry, M., and Lynch, G. The protease inhibitor leupeptin interferes with the development of LTP in hippocampal slices. *Brain Res.* **505:** 233-238, 1989.

2. Wang, Y., Zhu, G., Briz, V., Hsu, Y.-T., Bi, X. and Baudry, M. A molecular brake controls the magnitude of long-term potentiation. *Nature Communications* **5**, Article number: 3051; doi: 10.1038/ ncomms4051, 2014.
3. Liu, Y., Sun, J., Wang, Y., Lopez, D., Tran, J., Bi, X. and Baudry, M. Deleting both PHLPP1 and CANP1 rescues impairments in long-term potentiation and learning in both single knockout mice. *Learning & Memory* **23:** 399-404. 2016.
4. Zhu, G., Liu, Y., Wang, Y., Bi, X. and Baudry, M. Different patterns of electrical activity lead to long-term potentiation by activating different intracellular pathways. *J. Neurosci.* **35:** 621-633, 2015.
5. Liu, Y., Wang, Y., Zhu, G., Sun, J., Bi, X. and Baudry, M. A calpain-2 selective inhibitor enhances learning and memory by prolonging ERK activation. *Neuropharmacol.* 105: 471-477, 2016.
6. Luria, A.R. The mind of a mnemonist: A little book about a vast memory. Harvard University Press, Massachusetts and London, England. 1968.
7. Laurence Kim Peek (November 11, 1951 – December 19, 2009) was an American savant. Known as a "megasavant", he had an exceptional memory, but he also experienced social difficulties, possibly resulting from a developmental disability related to congenital brain abnormalities. He was the inspiration for the character Raymond Babbitt in the 1988 movie *Rain Man*. Although Peek was previously diagnosed with autism, he is now thought to have had FG syndrome.
8. Baudry, M. and Bi, X. Learning and memory: an emergent property of cell motility. *Neurobiol. Learning & Memory.* **104:**64-72, 2013.
9. Jacob, F. Evolution and Tinkering. *Science* 196: 1161-1166, 1977.
10. Wang, Y., Briz, V., Chishti, A., Bi, X. and Baudry, M. Distinct roles for μ- and m-calpain in synaptic NMDAR-mediated neuroprotection and extrasynaptic NMDAR-mediated neurodegeneration. *J. Neurosci.* **33:** 18880-18892, 2013.
11. Wang, Y., Hersheson, J., Lopez, D., Ben Hamad, M., Liu, Y., Lee, K.-H., Pinto, V., Seinfeld, J., Wiethoff, S., Sun, J,. Amouri, R.,

Hentati, F., Baudry, N., Tran, J., Singleton, A.B., Coutelier, M., Brice, A., Stevanin, G., Durr, A., Bi, X., Houlden, H. and Baudry, M. Defects in the *CAPN1* gene result in alterations in cerebellar development and in cerebellar ataxia in mice and humans. *Cell Reports* **16:** 79-91, 2016.

12. Forman, O.P., De Rision, L. and Mellersh, C.S. Missense mutation in CAPN1 is associated with spinocerebellar ataxia in the Parson Russell Terrier dog breed. Plos One. doi: 10.1371/journal.pone.0064627. Print 2013.
13. Baudry, M. and Bi, X. Calpain-1 and calpain-2: the yin and yang of synaptic plasticity and neurodegeneration. *Trends in Neurosciences* 2016 Feb 10. **39:** 235-245. pii: S0166-2236(16)00020-5. doi: 10.1016/j.tins.2016.01.007, 2016.

NOTES AND REFERENCES FOR CHAPTER 11

1. Wang, Y., Zhu, G., Briz, V., Hsu, Y.-T., Bi, X. and Baudry, M. A molecular brake controls the magnitude of long-term potentiation. *Nature Communications* **5**, Article number: 3051; doi: 10.1038/ ncomms4051, 2014.
2. Liu, Y., Wang, Y., Zhu, G., Sun, J., Bi, X. and Baudry, M. A calpain-2 selective inhibitor enhances learning and memory by prolonging ERK activation. *Neuropharmacol.* 105: 471-477, 2016.
3. Wang, Y., Lopez, D., Davey, P., Cameron D.J., Nguyen, K., Tran, J., Marquez, E., Liu, Y., Bi, X. and Baudry, M. Calpain-1 and calpain-2 play opposite roles in retinal ganglion cell degeneration induced by retinal ischemia/reperfusion injury. *Neurobiology of Disease* **93:** 121-128, 2016.
4. Wang, Y., Liu, Y., Lopez, D., Lee, M., Dayal, S., Hirtado, A., Bi, X. and Baudry, M. Protection against TBI-induced neuronal death with post-treatment with a selective calpain-2 inhibitor in mice. *J. Neurotrauma*, **34:** 1-13, 2018.
5. Wang, Y., Bi, X. and Baudry, M. To survive or to die: How neurons deal with it. In "Acute Neuronal Injury: The role of excitotoxic programmed cell death mechanisms." Denson Fujikawa (Ed), Springer Nature (Chapter 3), 2018.

6. Tsien, J.Z. Chapter 20: Cre-lox neurogenetics: History, Present and Future. In "Molecular-Genetic and Statistical Techniques for Behavioral and Neural Research." Academic Press. pp. 479-490. 2018.
7. Wang, Y., Liu, Y., Bi, X., Baudry, M. Calpain-1 and Calpain-2 in the Brain: New Evidence for a Critical Role of Calpain-2 in Neuronal Death. *Cells.* Dec 16;9(12):2698. doi: 10.3390/cells9122698.PMID: 33339205. 2020.
8. Woerman, A.L. et al. Tau prions from Alzheimer's disease and chronic traumatic encephalopathy patients propagate in cultured cells.... 113: E8187-E8196, 2016.
9. Wang, Y., Liu, Y., Nham, A., Sherbaf, A., Quach, D., Yahya, E., Ranburger, D., Bi, X., Baudry, M. Calpain-2 as a therapeutic target in repeated concussion-induced neuropathy and behavioral impairment. *Sci Adv.* Jul 1;6(27):eaba5547. doi: 10.1126/sciadv.aba5547. Print 2020 Jul. PMID: 32937436. 2020.

NOTES AND REFERENCES FOR CHAPTER 12

1. **Stereisomers.** Two molecules are described as stereoisomers if they are made of the same atoms connected in the same sequence, but the atoms are positioned differently in space. The difference between stereoisomers can only be seen when the three-dimensional arrangement of the molecules is considered. Optical isomers are molecules which are mirror images of one another. Often these mirror image molecules are referred to as **enantiomers.** Just as a right-handed glove cannot be superimposed on a left-handed glove, optical isomers cannot be superimposed on one another. Optical isomers can be described as left- or right-handed. Naturally occurring amino acids, the building blocks of life, are nearly all found in the left-handed state and produce left-handed proteins.

2. Chatterjee, P., Botello-Smith, W.M., Zhang, H., Qian, L., Alsamarah, A., Kent, D., Lacroix, J., Baudry, M. and Luo, Y. Can relative binding free energy predict selectivity of reversible covalent inhibitors? *J. Amer. Chem. Soc.,* 139: *179945-17952,* 2017.

3. **Selectivity versus potency.** Selectivity is the degree to which a drug acts on a given site relative to other sites. In other words, a very selective drug will only interact with a single target protein. Potency is an expression of the activity of a drug in terms of the concentration or amount of the drug required to produce a defined effect, whereas clinical efficacy judges the therapeutic effectiveness of the drug in humans. Although potency can be a good preclinical marker of the therapeutic potential of a drug, clinical efficacy should only be evaluated within the patient population using appropriate outcome measures.
4. Sanderson, K. Why sports concussions are worse for women. *Nature* 596: 26-28, 2021.
5. Baudry, M. et al. Identification and neuroprotective properties of NA-184, a calpain-2 inhibitor. *Pharmacol Res Perspect.* 2024 Apr;12(2):e1181. doi: 10.1002/prp2.1181.

NOTES AND REFERENCES FOR CHAPTER 13

1. https://www.fda.gov/drugs/types-applications/new-drug-application-nda
2. Nanosyn developed a synthesis schema, which requires 8 separate steps. The process was scaled up to produce about 180 g of NA-184.
3. https://www.fda.gov/drugs/pharmaceutical-quality-resources/current-good-manufacturing-practice-cgmp-regulations
4. https://www.healthline.com/health/what-is-dmso
5. Conceicao, J. et al. Cyclodextrins as drug carriers in pharmaceutical technology: the state of the art. *Curr. Pharm. Des.* 24: 1405-1433, 2018.
6. Singh, R.P. et al. Phospholipids: Unique carriers for drug delivery systems. *J. Drug Del. Sci. Tech.* 39: 166-179, 2017.
7. https://www.criver.com/products-services/discovery-services/integrated-drug-discovery?region=3601#:~:text=The%20industry%20standard%20timeline%20from,as%20little%20as%2024%20months.

NOTES AND REFERENCES FOR CHAPTER 14

1. https://www.cbinsights.com
2. Nordvang, E. Using protein biomarkers increases the chances of success in clinical trials. *Technology Networks, Proteomics & Metabolomics*, Jan 2020.
3. Shahim, P. et al. Neurofilament light as a biomarker in traumatic brain injury. *Neurology* 95: e610-e622, 2020.
4. Siman, R. et al. Serum SNTF, a Surrogate Marker of Axonal Injury, Is Prognostic for Lasting Brain Dysfunction in Mild TBI Treated in the Emergency Department. *Front. Neurology* 11:249. doi: 10.3389/fneur.2020.00249. 2020.
5. Wang, Y., Bradzionis, J., Dong, F., Patchana, T., Ghanchi, H., Podkovik, S., Wiginton, J.G., Marino, M., Duong, J., Wacker, M., Miulli, D.E., Neeki, M., Bi, X. and Baudry, M. P13BP, a calpain-2-mediated breakdown product of PTPN13, is a novel blood biomarker for traumatic brain injury. *J. Neurotrauma*. DOI: 10.1089/neu.2021.0229. 2021.

NOTES AND REFERENCES FOR CHAPTER 15

1. Gladwell, M. Outliers: The Story of Success. Little, Brown and Company; San Francisco, CA: 2008.
2. https://mantracare.org/ocd/ocd-examples/famous-scientists-with-ocd/
3. Baudry, M., Su, W. and Bi, X. The Calpain Proteolytic System. In Bradshaw Ralph A., Hart Gerald W. and Stahl Philip D. (eds.) *Encyclopedia of Cell Biology, Second Edition, vol. 1*, 2023, pp. 852–864. Oxford: Elsevier.
4. Dewitt, S. and Hallet, M.B. Calpain activation by calcium and its role in phagocytosis. *Adv. Exp. Med. Biol.* 1246:129-151, 2020.
5. Sato, T. et al. FAP-1 a protein phosphatase that associates with FAS. Science 268: 411-415, 1995.
6. Dutt, P. et al. m-Calpain is required for preimplantation embryonic development in mice. *BMC Dev. Biol.* 6: 3 doi: 10.1186/1471-213X-6-3, 2006.

7. Lon, H.K. et al. Pharmacokinetics, Safety, Tolerability, and Pharmacodynamics of Alicapistat, a Selective Inhibitor of Human Calpains 1 and 2 for the Treatment of Alzheimer Disease: An Overview of Phase 1 Studies. *Clin. Pharmacol. Drug Dev.* 8: 290-303. 2019.
8. Sattari, R. The ripple effects of funding on researchers and outputs. *Sci. Adv.* 8, eabb7348, 2022.
9. Van Dick, C.H. Lecanemab in early Alzheimer's disease. *N. Engl. J. Med.* 388:9-21, 2023.